PRACTICAL WAYS TO IMPROVE PATIENT ADHERENCE

Daniel J. Lewis

Steven R. Feldman, M.D., Ph.D.

Copyright © 2017 by Daniel J. Lewis and Steven R. Feldman
All rights reserved.

"I dedicate this book to my parents, Iona and Leonard Lewis, particularly my mother, who has sacrificed countless hours over the last 20 years as I have worked to perfect my writing skills. She will always be the greatest English teacher in my life. I also dedicate the book to my amazing academic mentors—Dr. Madeleine Duvic and Dr. Steven R. Feldman—for helping me develop my strong passion for dermatology, which I hope to continue building during my career."

— Daniel J. Lewis

"I dedicate this book to my incredible academic mentors, colleagues, research staff, research fellows, and patients, all of whom have contributed the ideas and sweat that have made my understanding of adherence what it is today. I also dedicate the book to my parents, Ed and Fran Feldman, who supported my early learning and career development, and my wife Leora Henkin, and our sons Jacob and Noah, who have taught me much about adherence and life over the years."

— Steven R. Feldman, M.D., Ph.D.

About the Authors

Daniel J. Lewis is a fourth-year M.D. student at Baylor College of Medicine and Research Assistant in the Department of Dermatology at The University of Texas MD Anderson Cancer Center in Houston, Texas. Dan earned a B.A. in Biology, *magna cum laude*, at the University of Pennsylvania. He is a member of the Alpha Omega Alpha Honor Medical Society. He has authored over 50 manuscripts in peer-reviewed journals, such as *Journal of the American Academy of Dermatology, JAMA Dermatology, Journal of Investigative Dermatology*, and *British Journal of Dermatology*. He has delivered many oral presentations, including one at the Late-Breaking Clinical Trials session of the 2017 American Academy of Dermatology Meeting. His chief professional interests are cutaneous T-cell lymphoma and psoriasis.

Dan also works as a professional sports journalist and has written over 80 articles for Yahoo! Sports, Bleacher Report, and SB Nation (www.DanielLewisSports.com). He also founded and served as Editor-in-Chief of *The Penn Sport Report*. Dan is also Founder and Co-President of Fitness for Life, a community service organization based in Philadelphia that seeks to combat the growing obesity epidemic in the United States by empowering children to live healthy lives.

Steven R. Feldman, M.D., Ph.D. is Professor of Dermatology, Pathology, and Social Sciences & Health Policy and Director of the Center for Dermatology Research at the Wake Forest University School of Medicine in Winston-Salem, North Carolina. He has authored over 800 peer-reviewed articles, and he has served as the principal investigator of industry, foundation, and federally funded studies.

Dr. Feldman has been ranked by ExpertScape as one of the top-five worldwide experts in psoriasis. He has served as a member of the medical board of the National Psoriasis Foundation, chaired that board's subcommittee on education, and served as Director of the Foundation's Chief Residents' Meeting on psoriasis treatment. He has also chaired the American Academy of Dermatology's Psoriasis Education Initiative Workgroup. He is the founder of www.DrScore.com and Chief Science Officer of Causa Research. He serves as the editor of or an editorial board member for five dermatology journals and is the author of *Compartments: How the Brightest, Best Trained, and Most Caring People Can Make Judgments That Are Completely and Utterly Wrong*. He is also the creator of *www.PromisedLandMuseum.org,* The Jewish Museum of the Palestinian Experience.

Table of Contents

About the Authors   3
Table of Contents   5
Chapter 1: Introduction   7

Section 1: The Problem of Poor Patient Adherence
Chapter 2: How Poor is Patient Adherence?   11
Chapter 3: Qualitative Measures of Adherence   18
Chapter 4: Clinical Studies on Adherence   27
Chapter 5: Why Is Adherence So Poor? It is Our Fault.   41
Chapter 6: A Pyramid Model for Improving Adherence   45

Section 2: Foundation – Trust and Accountability
Chapter 7: Establishing the Physician-Patient Relationship   49
Chapter 8: Setting the Right Office Visit Context   61
Chapter 9: Fostering Patient Accountability   66

Section 3: Practicality – Simplicity and Education
Chapter 10: Involving Patients in the Choice of Treatment   74
Chapter 11: Reducing the Burden of Treatment   83
Chapter 12: Educating and Providing Instructions   91
Chapter 13: Helping Patients Remember   103

Section 4: Psychology – Behavioral Techniques
Chapter 14: Anchoring   110
Chapter 15: Giving Salient Descriptions   115
Chapter 16: Emphasizing Losses Versus Gains   120
Chapter 17: Framing Risks of Side Effects   123
Chapter 18: Using Side Effects to Our Advantage   132

Section 5: Special Considerations

Chapter 19: Patients with Psychiatric Conditions	136
Chapter 20: Pediatric Patients	140
Chapter 21: Suddenly Adherent Patients	150
Chapter 22: The Most Adherence-Resistant Patients	152

Section 6: Sample Cases

Chapter 23: Pediatric Atopic Dermatitis	158
Chapter 24: Skin Cap for Psoriasis	163
Chapter 25: Coral Reef Psoriasis	169
Chapter 26: Scalp Psoriasis	172

Section 7: Final Thoughts

Chapter 27: Poor Adherence Is Not All Bad	180
Chapter 28: Conclusions	182

References	185

Chapter 1
Introduction

Have you ever encountered a patient with a common skin disorder who stated, "Doctor, you are the sixth dermatologist I have seen for my condition?" Perhaps this patient had a particularly resistant skin condition, an unusual disease variant that does not respond to treatment the way the condition usually does, or perhaps the skills of the previous dermatologists the patient had visited were questionable. But think about it for a moment—what is the chance that a patient could see five other dermatologists and not one of them make the correct diagnosis? That is pretty unlikely. And what is the chance that a patient could see five other dermatologists and not one of them prescribe the right treatment…even by chance? That is very unlikely too. There are so many caring, well-trained dermatologists, every one of whom would have made the right diagnosis and prescribed an appropriate treatment.

Still, it happens not infrequently that patients visit with that kind of story. What could be happening? Could patients with psoriasis somehow have inflammatory cells with mutated steroid receptors? Could patients be making antibodies against virtually every biologic therapy? Understanding how patients like these could fail treatment so many times is central to identifying the issues that contribute to treatment failure. Many patients who say, "Doctor, you are the sixth dermatologist I have seen for this," probably have one aspect in common that explains why their disease is so resistant to treatment. They probably are not using their medication as recommended.

The term "compliance" refers to how well patients use their medication. It is a term that was often taught in medical school, but it is now considered outdated and has largely been replaced with the term "adherence." "Compliance" suggests that patients should bow to an authoritarian doctor figure, whereas the "adherence" implies that patients actively engage in maintaining their health.

Poor adherence is ubiquitous in medicine and in dermatology in particular. The central thesis of this book is that we can improve our patients' treatment outcomes by getting them to use their medication better. Perhaps we can provide better patient care simply by encouraging patients to use the therapies we already have than we can by developing new ones. We may even be able to cure or clear patients of their disease with medications they have already tried—but did not use consistently or correctly—without resorting to riskier, more complicated, or costlier treatment regimens.

Providing quality medical care involves three key aspects: making the right diagnosis, prescribing the appropriate treatment, and getting patients to use their medication. While poor adherence is very common, current medical school and residency training curricula largely ignore adherence issues. They focus on the first two aspects of good medical care, the diagnosis and treatment, even though the latter two, the treatment and adherence, are more important in helping our patients get well. We learn about all sorts of pathologies and their respective treatments. Our pharmacology courses cover the absorption, distribution, and metabolism of drugs. But our training lacks a course that covers the principal factor that determines the variation in blood levels among patients. This variation is due, in large part, to variation in adherence—either how well or how poorly patients follow the treatment plans we recommend.

In Dr. Ben Barankin's book, *Dermographies: Autobiographies in Dermatology, Volume 2*, Dr. Stuart Maddin reported that his best piece of advice came from Dr. Marion Sulzberger, who "encouraged his residents to always be able to provide one further worthwhile treatment for the patient. He emphasized that having such depth was really the sign of a true consultant" (Barankin B, 2006). Perhaps it would have been better advice to suggest that to be a great consultant, one must always possess one additional technique to get patients to use their medication.

This book is not intended to present a detailed theoretical analysis of patients' adherence behavior, nor is it intended to provide a comprehensive review of adherence research. The objective of this book is to give you quick, practical tips to help you improve your patients' adherence and their treatment outcomes.

SECTION 1:
The Problem of Poor Adherence

Chapter 2: How Poor is Patient Adherence?

Chapter 3: Qualitative Measures of Adherence

Chapter 4: Clinical Studies on Adherence

Chapter 5: Why Is Adherence So Poor? It is Our Fault.

Chapter 6: A Pyramid Model for Improving Adherence

Chapter 2
How Poor is Patient Adherence?

Patients' adherence to treatment encompasses multiple steps. After we give patients a prescription (or send it directly to their pharmacy so they do not lose it), they may or may not fill the prescription. If they do, they may or may not start the treatment. If they start the treatment, they may use it well or poorly, and they may discontinue the treatment before they are supposed to do so. Primary adherence refers to whether they start the treatment; secondary adherence comprises those behaviors after initiating treatment.

Although research on adherence remains relatively limited in dermatology, other fields have studied it extensively while also assessing its impact on patient outcomes and identifying methods of improving patient adherence. Data on adherence to treatment for several non-dermatologic conditions—diabetes mellitus, sexually transmitted diseases, epilepsy, and asthma—provide a basis for understanding adherence in dermatology, which is likely worse than that seen in other fields of medicine.

Diabetes mellitus

Like many dermatologic conditions, diabetes mellitus is a

chronic disease that requires lifelong treatment. The pathogenesis of diabetes is well understood—it is a condition in which there is an absence of or resistance to insulin. Its diagnosis is also fairly straightforward, as there are specific laboratory testing criteria for its diagnosis. There are also several excellent treatments for the disease. For those patients who lack insulin, they can receive recombinant insulin injections. For patients who are resistant to insulin, diet, exercise, and medications can reduce the degree of insulin resistance. The main issue in treating diabetes involves getting patients to make the lifestyle modifications that these treatments require.

Diabetes, if uncontrolled, can lead to serious consequences—blindness, cardiovascular disease, neurologic disease, kidney failure, and even limb amputation. Considering these potentially horrible consequences, it would be logical to think that patients would adhere well to recommended treatment. However, the prevalence of uncontrolled diabetes demonstrates that patients can have a very serious disease with life-threatening consequences yet still not use treatment as recommended.

It is not enough for us to have medications to treat diabetes; we must also encourage patients to use them. We must counsel them, in an effective way, to incorporate taking their medication and monitoring their blood glucose into their daily routines. In this sense, the most important advances in the treatment of diabetes have focused on minimizing the burden of treatment. Superior delivery systems—insulin pens and pumps as well as long-acting treatments such as insulin glargine—and less invasive techniques to monitor blood glucose levels are innovations that facilitate proper patient management of diabetes. Dermatology patients might also benefit if these concepts were incorporated into the treatment of their skin disease. More broadly, all patients might benefit if these concepts were incorporated throughout medicine.

Another important lesson from the example of diabetes relates to disease assessment. Since diabetes involves elevated blood glucose levels, it would seem that measuring the blood glucose level in the doctor's office would be the number one way to assess the severity of disease. In reality, measuring blood glucose is a poor way to assess glucose control, as it only provides information about glucose levels at that very moment. It is very common for patients with diabetes to demonstrate excellent glucose control at the time of an office visit but not at other times, a very common phenomenon, one to which we will return and discuss in greater detail. Patients' behavior is substantially different preceding an office visit, affecting the severity of their illness when they are seen by the physician. In diabetes, measuring a hemoglobin A1C level, which provides a snapshot of the blood glucose level over a three-month period, allows the physician to assess glucose control between appointments.

Sexually transmitted infections

A common myth is that when patients have a symptomatic disease, one that bothers them a lot, they will adhere to treatment well. The care of patients with sexually transmitted diseases teaches us otherwise. Consider gonorrhea. One might assume that a patient with gonorrhea would want to get rid it as soon as possible. Theoretically, patients with gonorrhea should therefore be highly motivated to treat their disease given its stigma, its effects on their social behaviors, and the symptoms of a painful, purulent discharge. Gonorrhea could be treated effectively if patients would take an oral antibiotic twice a day for just one week. Yet patients with gonorrhea often fail to take the recommended oral antibiotic for even a single week. For this reason, gonorrhea is treated by administration of an intramuscular antibiotic. In dermatology, patients have symptomatic conditions that impair quality of life, but are they worse than "the clap?" The recommended treatment regimens in dermatology are typically far more complex and time-consuming than taking an oral antibiotic twice a day for one week. We cannot assume that just because patients have a severely symptomatic illness that they will adhere to treatment.

Skin diseases cause patients to experience significant suffering. Patients can develop intractable pruritus that interferes with sleep. The appearance of lesions, and the reactions of other people upon seeing the lesions, can be devastating to patients. One might assume that because skin disease is so distressing, dermatology patients would adhere to treatment. However, if patients with a condition as psychologically distressing as gonorrhea do not take their antibiotics for one week, how much worse is adherence in patients with chronic skin diseases who are receiving topical therapies? In one study of patients with moderate-to-severe psoriasis, the worse the impact of their disease, the *worse* their adherence. Patient adherence should not be taken for granted. If anything, we should assume that non-adherence is the norm and work assiduously to promote adherence.

Epilepsy

Epilepsy is another condition that requires lifelong treatment. Many effective anticonvulsant drugs are available. Yet it is often difficult, particularly in children with epilepsy, to maintain control of the disease. Even patients who appear to use their medication well, as evidenced by adequate blood levels of their antiepileptic medication, may experience breakthrough seizures.

Poor adherence may represent the primary cause of breakthrough seizures. Why would a patient with an adequate blood level of the antiepileptic medication develop breakthrough seizures? A drug blood level only reflects the level at the time of the office visit, which only reflects adherence in the days prior to the office visit. Just as patients with diabetes may exhibit adequate glucose control at the time of the office visit and inadequate control between visits, patients with epilepsy may take their medication regularly around the time of the office visit but not so regularly between visits. Drug blood levels provide information about adherence around the time the blood is drawn. Electronic adherence monitors would tell a different story—one of poor adherence between office visits.

Asthma

Adherence issues in treating children with asthma may be informative in treating children with atopic dermatitis and other conditions. Common strategies to optimize treatment outcomes have little to do with underlying genetic or immunologic issues. Fundamentally, both asthma and atopic dermatitis represent chronic diseases characterized by frequent flares. In both conditions, not only are there several treatments that may be prescribed at one time, but many of the treatments are very complex. Even worse, the various treatments that are used often require modification over time based on the ever-changing severity of the illness. The intricacies of treating these conditions is compounded by poor patient adherence.

Dr. Bruce Rubin, a pediatric pulmonologist, describes what asthma patients or their parents mean when they say, "My asthma medication is not working." (Rubin BK, 2004). With a few word substitutions, his descriptions would apply directly to children with atopic dermatitis. Although his classification scheme allows for the possibility of a physician making incorrect diagnosis or prescribing an inappropriate treatment, he recognizes poor adherence as the cause of poor treatment outcomes. Dr. Rubin's classification scheme emphasizes that there may be several reasons why patients do not use their medication:

1. The patient does not want to take medication—the patient is not actually sick, the patient is seeking secondary gain, or the medication is too expensive.
2. The patient does not understand how or when to use medication.
3. The patient is concerned about medication side effects.
4. The patient cannot feel the medication working.
5. The patient has unrealistic expectations.
6. The patient incorrectly thinks that they are inhaling medication.
7. The patient does not have asthma.
8. The patient needs an additional or stronger medication.

Notice that most of Dr. Rubin's reasons for poor adherence are patient-centered—a common way to frame the problem. However, a more practical way to frame the problem is as a physician-centered one, since we can control what we do. For example, the problem is not that our patients do not understand how or when to use medication; the problem is that we do not adequately communicate how and when to use the medication. We only have direct control over our own behavior, and so for us to solve the adherence problem, we have to change what we do.

Chapter 3
Qualitative Measures of Adherence

Obtaining an adherence history

Improving adherence in large part depends on being able to measure adherence. Unfortunately, there are very few accurate ways of assessing adherence in clinical practice. In general, the best approach might simply be to assume that our patients are not using their medication, especially when it is not working as well as we might have expected. We can attempt to obtain an adherence history, but patients will often report that they are taking their medication, even if they are not. These same patients might also tell their dentists they are flossing regularly even if they hardly floss at all.

Indirect questioning

It may be compelling to ask patients if they are following the treatment plan. However, it is best to avoid doing so in a way that challenges or condemns them. For example, while direct, it would be neither smart nor tactful to ask, "Are you drinking alcohol?" Too often, the patient will respond, "No," even if he or she is heavily drinking. Alternatively, we might ask, "How many cases of beer do you go through in a week?" In answering this question, the patient can proudly and honestly respond, "Doctor, I only drink a few beers on the weekend."

When asking whether patients have been taking their medication, consider instead asking how often they have not. We might ask, "How often do you miss doses? Every day or every other day?" This question frames missing occasional doses as acceptable, encouraging patients to be honest about their adherence. It also makes them feel proud of themselves when they can report missing a dose only once a week. Conversely, asking, "Have you been taking the medication?" leads patients into reflexively answering, "Yes, doctor."

> **Recommended quote:**
> We should avoid asking, *"Have you been taking the medication?"* We are more likely to get an honest answer if we instead ask, *"How often do you miss doses? Every day or every other day?"*

This method, known as "indirect questioning," may lead to more accurate responses about adherence. Below are additional indirect, non-judgmental questions we can ask to evaluate our patients' adherence (Alinia H, 2014):

Adherence assessment questionnaire

1. Do you need a refill?
    - Yes
    - No
2. When you need a refill:
    - I call the pharmacy

- I go by the pharmacy
- I use an online or other electronic refill system
- Not applicable

3. If it is time for a refill and you still have extra medicine:
   - I wait to fill the refill
   - I fill the refill anyway
   - I throw the old medicine away and get the refill
   - Not applicable

4. Does the pharmacy send you medication even when you don't need it?
   - Yes
   - No
   - Not applicable

5. Where do you keep extra (prescribed) medicine that has accumulated?
   - In the medicine cabinet
   - In the kitchen
   - In another room or location
   - I dispose of extra medicine
   - Not applicable

6. I do the following with extra medicine I have accumulated (circle all that apply):
   - Return it to the pharmacy
   - Donate it to charitable organizations
   - Share it with friends and relatives
   - Dispose of it
   - Not applicable

7. I usually dispose of unused medicine:
   - Down the sink

- Down the toilet
- In the trash can
- Not applicable

8. Do you keep extra syringes of medication refrigerated?
   - Yes
   - No
   - Not applicable
9. Is the cabinet where you keep extra medicine locked?
   - Yes
   - No
   - Not applicable

The adherent patient would respond "not applicable" to these questions; most patients would give some other response.

There are some patients who are incredibly convincing in their prostrations about their near-perfect adherence to treatment. When therapy is not working as well as expected, it may be best to trust patients yet still consider the possibility of poor use of the medication. The Cold War "Trust, but verify" advice may be apropos.

Religiosity and honesty

Researchers such as Dan Ariely who have studied honesty have found that individuals are generally more honest when they are placed in a religious frame of mind. Students cheated less on examinations after they were first asked to list as many of the Ten Commandments as they could. It did not matter how many they listed, how many they got correct, or even if they were religious at all. Simply making them think about religion caused them to be more honest. Therefore, when we are caring for patients who we know are religious, priming them by first asking them about their church, mosque, or synagogue may yield more honest answers when we then ask them about their use of their medication.

Informal auditing

For patients using self-administered biologics for psoriasis, we can deftly assess adherence by asking, "Are you keeping the extra injectors you have accumulated in the refrigerator like you are supposed to?" The correct answer is "Doctor, I am not really sure what you are talking about. I do not have any extra syringes." If patients instead respond affirmatively, we immediately know they are accumulating extras and not using the medication as prescribed.

> **Recommended quote:**
> For patients on biologics, we can assess adherence by asking, *"Are you keeping the extra injectors you have accumulated in the refrigerator like you are supposed to?"*

Dr. Keith Vaughan of University Place, Washington suggests advising patients to bring their current medication regimen to their follow-up visit as part of an informal auditing process. This strategy is particularly helpful if we prescribed multiple medications at the initial visit or if we might expect adherence issues based on their demeanor or overall behavior. In reality, though, we should anticipate adherence issues at every visit.

Tube weights and pill counts

In research studies assessing adherence to topical therapy, we can weigh the medication tubes. This method is not practical for everyday practice, but we can still assess patient adherence simply by looking at the medication. We can count pills or look at the tubes and clearly recognize that patients are not using the medication if the tube or bottle remains full. However, an empty tube or bottle does not necessarily mean patients used the medication; they may have simply squeezed or poured it into their trashcan at home.

Similarly, pill counts may be unreliable. If we want to assess adherence by using pill counts, we should not give patients 60 pills for twice-daily use and suggest that they return in one month. If we do, an empty bottle might mean they either exhibited perfect adherence or threw out the pills. In one study using electronic monitors, a patient returned with an empty bottle and a self-recorded treatment diary indicating that she had taken the medication daily as prescribed (Krejci-Manwaring J, 2007). The electronic monitor showed that, in reality, she had only opened the bottle once, presumably to toss the pills into the trashcan.

We can make pill counts more useful by prescribing more pills than patients would actually need. For example, we might prescribe 70 pills for twice-a-day use for one month. If patients present an empty bottle at the return visit, then they likely threw the pills in the trashcan. Meanwhile, if the bottle contains 10 pills, then they almost certainly must be using their medication very well.

Electronic monitoring

Electronic monitors represent an excellent resource for assessing adherence. WestRock Corporation's Medication Event Monitoring System (MEMS) bottle caps record the date and time each time the medication bottle is opened **(Figure 1)**. Although these devices are very practical for clinical research studies, they are costly and not practical for everyday clinic use.

Figure 1: Electronically monitored bottle caps. The WestRock Corporation's Medication Event Monitoring System (MEMS) bottle caps can provide detailed and objective information on how often patients use their medication.

Adherence survey studies in dermatology

Before the development of electronic monitors, adherence in dermatology had been measured primarily via surveys. One survey asked patients with psoriasis how well they had been using their medication. The survey was anonymous, so patients should have felt comfortable providing an honest report. Nearly 40% admitted to not using their medication as directed (Richards HL, 1999); we suspect most of the other 60% were not telling the truth. A similar survey assessing the use of topical steroids for psoriasis also found that 40% of subjects reported poor adherence (Brown KK, 2006). Frustrations related to efficacy and inconvenience as well as a fear of side effects were among the most common reasons they did not use their medication. Other factors included costs, unclear instructions, overly complicated directions, and the unpleasant feeling of the medication.

Since Denmark maintains a national pharmacy database, researchers in Denmark can assess how long patients take to fill their prescriptions, if they fill them at all. In one Danish study, dermatologists had written prescriptions for medications to treat patients with various skin diseases—acne, atopic dermatitis, infections, and psoriasis (Storm A 2008). The researchers found that 90% of prescriptions for acne and skin infections were filled within one month; many people think that sounds good, but it is far from a six-sigma level of quality—if only 90% of Toyota® cars worked, we would be far from satisfied. For atopic dermatitis, only two-thirds were filled, and for psoriasis, only half of the prescriptions were filled!

Psoriasis varies in its severity and its effects on patients' lives. We might assume that patients with severe psoriasis would try the hardest to reduce their suffering from the disease. Nevertheless, surveys found that patients with severe disease—as measured by disease involvement or its impact on quality of life—were less likely to adhere to treatment than those with mild disease (Zaghloul SS, 2004). Perhaps the brain does not want to think about severe disease or treatment of it. In short, adherence can be highly unpredictable, and we should avoid making conjectures about adherence without testing our predictions.

Chapter 4
Clinical Studies on Adherence

Assessing patient adherence—whether by pill counts or patient-reported treatment diaries—poses significant limitations. Patients often report having used far more medication than they actually used. Pill counts and tube weights are similarly unreliable because patients may have dumped the medication into their trashcan at home. On the other hand, electronic monitoring devices—used in patients with HIV infection, diabetes, epilepsy, and asthma—offer a more accurate, objective method of assessing adherence. They, too, show that adherence is less than what patients self-report. Adherence studies done in dermatology show similar findings.

Psoriasis

Psoriasis is a chronic disease that can frustrate both us and our patients. Finding a sufficiently effective therapy can be difficult, and our treatments seem to lose efficacy over time. Some of the earliest adherence research in dermatology involved patients with psoriasis. One early study assessed patients' use of 6% salicylic acid gel, which was administered in an attempt to potentiate the effects of 0.1% Protopic® (tacrolimus) ointment (Carroll CL, 2005). Topical tacrolimus is effective in treating psoriasis affecting the face or intertriginous areas, and perhaps topical tacrolimus might also be effective in treating plaque psoriasis in other areas if combination use with salicylic acid were to promote greater penetration.

In the study, subjects were given tacrolimus ointment to apply to their lesions on both sides of the body for eight weeks. They were also instructed to apply salicylic acid gel twice a day to their plaques—but to use it only on one side of the body, allowing for left-right comparisons. The salicylic acid was provided in containers equipped with electronic monitors. Subjects were informed that they were being monitored and were asked to maintain a medication diary and bring their medication bottles to clinic for weighing. However, they were not told about the electronic monitors in the medication bottle caps.

The use of electronic monitors opened a window into the previously unseen aspects of patient adherence in the treatment of psoriasis. Some patients used the salicylic acid nearly as we had recommended. One particularly obsessive-compulsive patient documented using it exactly as the electronic monitor indicated (Balkrishnan R, 2003). Other patients did not use it nearly as well. Two subjects reported using it as directed but used it rarely according to the monitors. One subject, despite opening the container only once, presented to clinic complaining of symptoms of salicylism. Based on these findings, we can only wonder how much more effective drugs might be in clinical trials if subjects used them more reliably.

Figure 2: Weekly use of 6% salicylic acid gel in combination with 0.1% tacrolimus ointment in patients with psoriasis. The electronically monitored bottle caps showed that patients used their medication less often than they had indicated in their diary. Interestingly, use of the medication decreased by 20% every five weeks; the decreasing use of medication over time likely leads to loss of efficacy, a phenomenon often interpreted clinically as "tachyphylaxis." Abbreviations: MEMS, Medication Event Monitoring System.

According to the treatment diaries, subjects applied the salicylic acid more than 90% of the time over the eight-week study period **(Figure 2)**. However, according to the electronic monitors, they used it on the first day, and then their use declined dramatically, by about 40%, over the next few days (Carroll CL, 2004). Adherence continued to decrease slowly over time, aside from brief increases occurring at two-week intervals. What accounted for these regular increases? The study visits. Just as individuals tend to floss their teeth more often just before seeing the dentist, patients use their medications in the days before they come to see us. The adherence literature terms this "white coat compliance," but we prefer to call it "the dental floss phenomenon."

In the salicylic acid study, adherence decreased by 20% every five weeks. Although the study only lasted eight weeks, we can extrapolate from the data that adherence would reach zero after 25 weeks, or after about six months, if adherence were to continue to decrease at the observed rate beyond this eight-week study (it is a common error to extrapolate beyond the range of the data, but we do so here for illustrative purposes). In dermatology, we have assigned a name to the outcome that results when adherence to topical therapy approaches zero. We call it "tachyphylaxis." Traditionally, tachyphylaxis is thought to be, "The more you use the steroid, the less it works," potentially due to a downregulation of steroid receptors. But actually, tachyphylaxis is, "The *less* you use the steroid, the less it works." Before this study, dermatologists were unaware of how patients actually used their medication, and so we simply believed patients when they claimed, "Doctor, I have been using the medication religiously. It just does not work anymore."

One way we could prove that tachyphylaxis is due to poor adherence would be to conduct a study in which we gave triamcinolone to patients with localized plaque psoriasis. We could give them the medication in blue bottles equipped with electronic monitors. Then when the medication inevitably stopped working, we could administer the same medication in red bottles and demonstrate that it started working again. But we already do something similar in our practices. When patients develop "tachyphylaxis," we often switch to another steroid of the same class. If tachyphylaxis were due to the downregulation of steroid receptors, when one mid-potency steroid stopped working, the others would not work either (Ali SM, 2007).

Atopic dermatitis

Atopic dermatitis is another condition that is often complicated by poor patient adherence. For example, consider a child with horrific, lichenified lesions affecting the entire body that are refractory to all sorts of outpatient therapies. If we were to admit this child to the hospital and treat him or her with topical 0.1% triamcinolone ointment— perhaps along with anti-staphylococcal antibiotics, if indicated—the lesions would clear almost completely in just two or three days. Hospitalization would lead to rapid improvement not because it removes the patient from the dust mites at home or somehow reduces stress, but rather because it simply ensures that the triamcinolone is applied.

A "real life" trial assessed adherence to topical triamcinolone in children with atopic dermatitis (Krejci-Manwaring J, 2007). Patients and their parents were given 0.1% triamcinolone ointment and were instructed to use it twice a day. The medication was provided in bottles equipped with electronic monitors. They were told to return in one month. They were not told about the electronic monitors. To understand what adherence is like in "real life," they were not even told they were part of a study!

We learned from the adherence study on psoriasis that patients do not use their topical medications very well. We have to wonder how much worse adherence is in real-life clinical practice than it was in the research study. The psoriasis study included a number of factors—patients knowing that they were being monitored, filling out treatment diaries, coming in for return visits every two weeks, receiving written instructions, and being compensated for their participation—that should have motivated the study subjects to use their medication better than they would in everyday practice. Accordingly, in order to understand patient adherence outside of a formal research study, unlike in the psoriasis study, patients in this "real life" atopic dermatitis study were not told that they were part of a trial. There was no consent form. If the patients had known that they were part of a study, it might have affected their behavior, a principle known as the Hawthorne effect (Davis SA, 2013).

In the study, use of the triamcinolone was excellent on the first day **(Figure 3)**. However, over the next three days, adherence dropped by 60-70%. It continued to decrease over time, but then it suddenly increased at one month—at the time of the return office visit.

Poor adherence in children with atopic dermatitis should not be surprising. In treating pediatric patients, there are now multiple parties who can contribute to poor adherence: the child and caregivers. If you have ever tried putting sunscreen or a topical medication on your child, you understand why adherence is often so poor in pediatric patients.

Figure 3: Daily use of 0.1% triamcinolone ointment in children with atopic dermatitis. Although patients used the triamcinolone ointment on the first day of the study, adherence plummeted over the next two days and then continued to decrease. The rate at which adherence declines likely correlates with the rate at which "tachyphylaxis" develops.

An open-label study was performed in children with atopic dermatitis to evaluate whether measures aimed at improving adherence would yield better treatment outcomes (Yentzer BA, 2010). The study participants were given Desonate® (desonide) gel, a low-potency, easy-to-apply steroid. They also received written instructions to help them understand the medication. Subjects were told that they were being given a "cortisone-type" medication, without mentioning the word "steroid." In addition to scheduling a return visit in one week, patients were contacted three days after they began treatment to inquire about their use of the medication.

The interventions worked well. Patients reported a high degree of satisfaction with the aqueous gel vehicle. Moreover, whereas in the previous study use of the triamcinolone ointment decreased by 60-70% within three days, use of the desonide gel in this study decreased by only 30% in the first week and was roughly 50% at the end of four weeks. Nearly all subjects demonstrated significant improvement; mean Eczema Area and Severity Index (EASI) scores improved from baseline by approximately 60%.

One pediatric dermatology expert reported that for patients with treatment-resistant atopic dermatitis, he is not afraid to use ultra potent topical steroids, add penetration enhancers, recommend wet wraps, or switch to potent systemic agents such as methotrexate or cyclosporine. How effective are these approaches when the mother is afraid to use low-to-medium-potency topical steroids? Can we expect her to apply an ultra potent steroid if she was afraid of using a weaker one? Will she apply two medications or use wet wraps after she was reluctant or unable to use even one medication regularly? For disease that is "resistant" to treatment, we do not need to resort to higher potency steroids or more complicated treatment regimens. Simply getting patients to use their medication better, even a modestly potent topical steroid, can be very effective.

Hand dermatitis

Applying a topical agent is generally more difficult than taking a pill. One study examined the use of tacrolimus ointment as maintenance therapy for hand dermatitis in patients who had received a three-week course of oral prednisone (Krejci-Manwaring J, 2006). Both the bottles containing the prednisone pills and the containers filled with tacrolimus ointment were equipped with electronic monitors. Patients were instructed to take the oral prednisone once daily for three weeks and apply the tacrolimus ointment twice daily for 12 weeks.

Use of the oral prednisone was generally good; overall, patients missed only a few doses. Use of the tacrolimus ointment, though, was worse and declined over the 12 weeks of treatment. Of note, patients appeared to use the topical treatment more frequently on the day of the visit in addition to a few days before and after the visit **(Figure 4)**.

Assessments of the average adherence of the entire study group do not reveal the variation in adherence among subjects; adherence in individual patients varied tremendously. One subject opened the prednisone bottle only a single time, presumably to toss the pills into the trashcan, as she returned with an empty bottle (Krejci-Manwaring J, 2007). Another patient, who had developed hand dermatitis due to obsessive hand washing, was also obsessive in using her tacrolimus ointment, applying it eight to 14 times per day. In short, it is very difficult to predict how individual patients will use their medication; the potential range in behavior, from underuse to overuse, is enormous.

Figure 4: Medication use varies in relation to follow-up visits. Patients' use of 6% salicylic acid gel for psoriasis and tacrolimus ointment for hand dermatitis was seemingly erratic. The percentage of patients who use their medication on a given day was plotted in relation to the day of the most recent or upcoming follow-up visit. Patients appeared to use their medication on the day of the visit in addition to few days before and after the visit. They were far less likely to use their medication when there was no recent or upcoming follow-up visit.

Acne

Although teenagers may be very bothered by their acne, they are not entirely adherent to treatment; not even close! After all, teenagers are particularly poor at seeking delayed gratification, and they may quickly give up on medications that do not produce rapid improvement.

In one study, teenagers with acne were given Differin® (adapalene) 0.1% gel in tubes equipped with electronic monitors (Yentzer BA, 2011). The study objective was to assess their adherence and evaluate interventions to improve their adherence. The study involved 60 patients, and all were instructed to apply the adapalene once daily for 12 weeks. One group—the standard-of-care group—was re-evaluated at six weeks and at 12 weeks. Another group—the frequent visit group—returned at one week, two weeks, four weeks, six weeks, eight weeks, and 12 weeks. This schedule was designed to mirror follow-up intervals in a standard clinical trial, with the hypothesis that additional visits would promote better adherence. A third group—the electronic reminder group—received a daily phone call to remind them to use their medication. The fourth group—the parental reminder group—consisted of patients whose parents were called daily and were asked to remind the teen daily to use their medication.

In the standard-of-care group, adherence began at about 70% before decreasing to 40% over the course of the study **(Figure 5)**. As expected, the frequent-visit group displayed the highest adherence, starting at about 80% before dropping to around 50% at the end of the study. The phone call reminders to the teenagers seemed to accomplish little; patients receiving these reminders exhibited adherence similar to that of the standard-of-care group. Interestingly, the parental reminder group showed the *worst* adherence of

Figure 5: Weekly use of Differin® (adapalene) gel associated with various interventions in teenagers with acne. Patients were treated with adapalene gel daily for 12 weeks and divided into four groups based on the intervention they received to promote adherence. Frequent visits produced the highest level of adherence. Daily electronic reminders had little effect on adherence compared to the standard of care. Parental reminders yielded the worst adherence.

Actinic keratosis

Adherence is abysmal in children with atopic dermatitis, teenagers with acne, and young adults with psoriasis. How is adherence in older patients? In one study, patients with actinic keratoses were given 0.5% Carac® (fluorouracil) cream and were instructed to apply it daily for four weeks (Yentzer BA, 2009). They were also asked to complete a daily treatment diary and bring the medication to clinic for weighing. They were informed that they would be monitored but not that there were electronic monitors in the medication container caps. In contrast to the previous studies assessing adherence in psoriasis, atopic dermatitis, hand dermatitis, and acne, adherence in this study was excellent. Roughly 90% of subjects were adherent, taking at least 80% of the number of recommended doses. In fact, on many occasions, when subjects missed a dose on one day, they used the medication twice the next day to make up for the missed dose.

5-flurouracil is very irritating; one might have predicted that adherence would have been terrible because of the potential for irritation. On the contrary, excellent adherence was observed. Several factors might explain the high level of adherence observed in this study. First, the duration of treatment was shorter than in the other studies, thus making adherence over the entire study period more feasible. Second, while we might think that patients would not use agents that cause irritation, the irritation might actually act as a constant reminder to use the medication, resulting in better adherence. The irritation may also make patients think the medication is working, thereby encouraging them to continue. It is also possible that the nature of the disease drove adherence, as actinic keratoses are considered pre-cancerous lesions, and patients may be motivated by a fear of cancer. However, this possibility is not particularly likely, as motivation to get well does not seem to be a very good driver of adherence. Most importantly, though, perhaps older patients are simply more adherent than their younger counterparts. Older patients may be used to taking medications and may already have systems in place that remind them to do so.

Chapter 5
Why Is Adherence So Poor? It is Our Fault.

Adherence researchers continue to wrestle with the question, "Why is patient adherence so poor?" There are a number of factors that are thought to contribute to poor adherence. Understanding potential barriers to adherence can help guide us in implementing strategies to help our patients use their medication.

Blame ourselves, not our patients

Our healthcare system in the U.S. is holding us increasingly responsible for our patients' outcomes. On one hand, working to give our patients the best possible outcome is what we want and expect from ourselves. On the other hand, we may wonder why we are held responsible when our patients are simply not using their medication.

It is perfectly reasonable for us to be held accountable for our patients' outcomes. Not only must we make the right diagnosis and prescribe the right treatment, but we must also encourage patients to use their medication. Poor adherence is largely a *physician* problem, not a patient problem. While many physicians might disagree with this construct, holding ourselves responsible for poor adherence actually does us a service, as it is easier for us to change ourselves than it is to change our patients.

Much of the research on adherence has focused on how patient-related issues contribute to poor adherence. However, this perspective does not adequately describe our role in ensuring adherence. Attributing poor adherence to patients' lack of understanding, for example, undersells our responsibility for conveying critical information in an effective manner. We can redefine several common patient barriers to adherence as physician or health system hurdles **(Table 1)** (Devine F, 2017).

Patient barriers to adherence	Physician or health system hurdles
Health literacy Education level Lack of knowledge of medication Concern about side effects	Inadequate transmission of information about condition or medication
Beliefs about medication Stigma or need for secrecy Cultural beliefs	Inadequate attention to aligning treatment with patient's beliefs and culture
View of symptoms ("Felt good, so did not take medication")	Inadequate education about need for treatment of asymptomatic disease
Medication abuse	Inadequate effort in addressing patient's substance abuse
Forgetting to take medication	Inadequate effort in helping patient set up reminder systems
Depression leading to poor motivation to take medication	Inadequate effort in identifying or addressing patient's depression

Cost and lack of insurance coverage	Prescribing unaffordable medications
Lack of caregiver	Inadequate attention to patient's support system
Lack of access to healthcare and resources	Inadequate provision of service at patient's location
Busy, competing priorities Changes to routine	Inadequate attention to patient's schedule when prescribing medication
Pill burden Complicated treatment regimen	Prescribing overly complex treatment regimens involving too many medications and a too frequent dosing schedule

Table 1: Common barriers to patient adherence redefined as physician or health system hurdles

We must recognize that while it is easy for us to write prescriptions, it is much harder for our patients to use the medications we prescribe. We must help them overcome a number of obstacles before they can successfully use their medication. In dermatology, we often prescribe topical agents, which require a higher level of dedication and precision, and so it is far harder for us to get our patients to adhere to treatment than it is for physicians in other fields.

There are some factors affecting adherence that remain out of our control. For instance, patients who are seeking disability may actively work to ensure that their condition does not improve. Nevertheless, there are many factors that we can control. As described in Chapter 9: Fostering Patient Accountability, the standard approach for getting patients to take medication is a model for failure. We can do better. The ensuing chapters describe practical ways for us to improve patient adherence.

Chapter 6
A Pyramid Model for Improving Adherence

There are many reasons why patients do not use their medication. Some adherence researchers argue that we must target our approach for improving adherence in an individual patient to the specific reason why he or she is non-adherent. While this method may work, a more general approach may be effective. We can apply some general principles to encourage all patients to use their medication, regardless of their reason for not using it.

The three levels for improving patient adherence are illustrated in the pyramid below **(Figure 6)**: (1) building a strong foundation centered on trust and accountability, (2) addressing practical issues to make treatment as easy as possible for our patients, and (3) utilizing specific behavioral techniques to give our patients an additional nudge to use their medication.

The first step in improving adherence entails building a foundation that fosters trust. Patients are cynical of insurance companies and the pharmaceutical industry; therefore, they must trust us before they will trust the medication we prescribe. Our patients will trust us only if they realize we care about them. We care about our patients, but the fact that we care about them has no impact on their behavior. None! Their behavior is determined solely by their *perception* of whether or not we care about them. Promoting trust and a sense that we care about them is determined by how we act and the context in which they see us act.

Once we establish a strong social bond with our patients, they will not want to let us down. Instead of fearing the medication, they may fear the embarrassment of not meeting the expectations of a physician who cares about them. Holding them accountable for the use of their medication—for example, with an office visit to see how well the treatment is working—is another component of the foundation on which adherence is built.

Psychology: Behavioral Techniques — Giving patients an extra "nudge" using behavioral strategies

Practicality: Simplicity and Education — Reducing the burden of treatment

Foundation: Trust and Accountability — Establishing the physician-patient relationship

Figure 6: A pyramid model for improving adherence. The first step entails building a foundation centered on trust and accountability. The second step involves addressing practical issues to make the treatment process as easy as possible for patients. The final step involves employing practical psychological techniques to give patients an extra "nudge" to use their medication.

The second level involves making the treatment process as easy as possible for our patients. For one, we should always attempt to prescribe low-cost and fast-acting medications; combination drugs may be useful to simplify the treatment regimen for certain diseases. We can shorten the initial treatment interval to make the apparent burden of treatment appear lighter. Providing written instructions and suggesting medication reminders are other simple measures that will empower patients to use their medication.

The final level involves utilizing specific psychological techniques that encourage patients to follow their medication regimen. For example, recognizing that many patients exhibit an unreasonable fear of rare side effects, we can frame the risks of therapies in ways that put those risks into a more accurate perspective. In addition, a technique known as "anchoring," can make our patients less concerned about the burden of treatment. We can also use side effects to our advantage, proactively advising patients that a potential side effect is "a sign that the drug is working." By using these behavioral strategies, we can give patients a strong "nudge" to use their medication.

SECTION 2:
Foundation — Trust and Accountability

Chapter 7: Establishing the Physician-Patient Relationship

Chapter 8: Setting the Right Office Visit Context

Chapter 9: Fostering Patient Accountability

Chapter 7
Establishing the Physician-Patient Relationship

We are caring, but we have to show it.

Medicine, at its heart, is a "people" business. We are not laboratory technicians following standardized protocols involving fixed quantities of highly purified reagents. It would seem that making accurate diagnoses and prescribing the appropriate treatment would be enough to help patients get well, but such is not the case.

While these duties are very important, we need to do more to be effective caregivers. We must also convey a sense of caring and trust. This aspect comes naturally for some doctors, whereas others do it with showmanship. There is nothing wrong with either approach. The key is to recognize the need for a strong doctor-patient relationship and work toward building one. If patients feel that we do not care and that they cannot trust us, they are not going to use the medications we prescribe, and they are not going to get well.

Some doctors may feel that their relationships with patients are their *raison d'être* for being doctors. However, for the rest of us, establishing a strong physician-patient relationship has a practical purpose. If we cultivate one, patients are more likely to use their medication; if we do not, they are less likely to do so. "Touchy feely" doctors are able to establish a close, interpersonal relationship with patients. For practical purposes, though, we do not have to be "touchy feely" doctors for patients to view us as their ally. We just need to exhibit some of the behaviors that come naturally to the physician-humanist.

Vic Marks provides some excellent techniques in his article, "Service Excellence in Dermatology" **(Table 2)** (Marks VJ, 2004).

First impressions count	Look patients in the eye when you meet them. Introduce yourself in an appropriate manner. Even before they meet you, make sure your front office communicates the right message.
Let patients tell you their story	Do not interrupt if you can help it. Do not appear rushed.
Show you are listening	Look intently while patients speak. Ask questions to show your understanding. Restate what they say.
Touch their skin	Touching helps communicate a thorough examination was done. Using a lighted magnifying device such as a dermatoscope helps in this regard.
Explain the condition and the reason for treatment	Use understandable terminology.
Show empathy	Say something such as "your previous treatments have probably been frustrating."

Address psychosocial issues	Recommend support groups.
Solicit input and questions	Ask "do you have any other questions?" before ending the visit
Make yourself accessible	Give your contact information to patients. Make sure there are appropriate policies in place in case patients have questions or concerns after the visit.

Table 2: Service excellence skills: showing we care

As Marks outlines, for patients who say they have taken several medications but still have active disease, we can empathize, "I bet the previous treatments have been very frustrating, right?"

> **Recommended quote:**
> To show empathy for our patients, we can ask, *"I bet the previous treatments have been very frustrating, right?"*

These words are very powerful. The patient will think we have read their mind, but in fact patients are almost always frustrated by the previous treatment; if they had a treatment they liked that worked very well, they would not be sitting on our examination table with active disease.

Physical examination

One measure to ensure that patients trust us is to demonstrate that a thorough examination was performed. Conducting a complete skin examination in patients who are willing to have one done is prudent. It may help to provide a written brochure on skin examination to inform patients why we are asking to do the full examination. Touching the areas being examined helps us communicate to patients that we performed a thorough exam. When examining the back, the patient cannot tell what was or was not examined, so it may help to palpate the back as we look at it so that the patient knows what parts were evaluated. When a patient points to a pigmented lesion and says, "This one is different from all my other spots. It has changed, and I am worried about it," we will almost undoubtedly need to perform a biopsy; even if it looks like a seborrheic keratosis, it might be an atypical melanoma. But before we perform the biopsy, we should nevertheless examine the lesion carefully using a lighted magnifying glass, such as a dermatoscope. Using such a device will likely not affect whether or not a biopsy is necessary, but it will help the patient realize that we carefully examined the lesion.

In describing the craft of magic, Henning Nelms wrote, "As the object of the effect is to convince the spectators, their interpretation of the evidence is the only thing that counts. When the effect consists in taking a cannon ball from an empty hat, the audience must believe that the hat is empty and that the cannon ball is heavy. If the spectators accept this, a one-ounce half-globe of papier-mâché is as good as a twenty-pound iron sphere; if they regard the ball as an imitation, iron is no better than papier-mâché" (Nelms H, 1969). However, medicine is not magic. Whereas a magician does not need to produce an iron ball, doctors do need to make the right diagnosis and prescribe the right treatment. But if patients are not convinced of as much, they will be left feeling as unsatisfied as the audience watching a magician who does produce an iron ball but does not convince the audience of it.

Hand washing

The spread of methicillin-resistant *Staphylococcus aureus* (MRSA) is a growing problem in the U.S. We are told to wash our hands to help prevent the spread of the bacteria. Patients expect us to do it. If we wash our hands in the hallway and the patients do not see us do it, they might think we are an infectious menace.

One dermatologist, Dr. W. Lee Davis, of Chambersburg, Pennsylvania, says that after washing and drying his hands, he carries the used paper towels into the exam room and disposes of them in there, letting the patient see that he just finished washing his hands. What a wonderful, practical way of making sure our patients witness a quality effort we do that might otherwise go unseen and unappreciated.

Even better, we can help ensure our patients remember that we washed our hands by saying, "Let me use the alcohol here to protect you from flesh-eating bacteria, Ebola, MRSA, and the other evil humours of the medical office." Describing these scary bugs paints an unforgettable image in patients' minds, an example of the concept

> **Recommended quote:**
> To help our patients remember that we washed our hands, we can say, "Let me use the alcohol here to protect you from flesh-eating bacteria, Ebola, MRSA, and the other evil humours of the medical office."

of salience, which is discussed further in Chapter 15: Giving Salient Descriptions.

Facial expressions and body language

Patients are silent observers of our face and body language. They might recall a single discouraging statement or inappropriate facial expression that we made. These actions might negatively influence their opinion of us, even though our knowledge or bedside manner might be stellar. Thus, communication skills are often more important than the diagnosis itself.

Speech characteristics such as rate, loudness, pitch, and pauses also affect patients' perceptions of us. Non-verbal cues influence patients more often than verbal information. A blank expression is unwelcoming, as it communicates disinterest and a lack of empathy. Nodding our heads, making eye contact, leaning forward, and smiling are all positive gestures that show attentiveness and are often well received. Similarly, praising patients for taking the initiative to come to clinic also helps build rapport, especially when we consider that they often have to adjust their schedule to leave work or school to see us during normal clinic hours.

Timeliness

Showing up on time for clinic is *de rigueur*. In addition, when opening the door to the examination room to see a patient, open it slowly; if we rush in, the patient will think we are in a hurry. Similarly, we must avoid looking at our watches when we are with patients. Instead, we can place a clock on the wall directly behind the patient so that when when we look at the time, the patient thinks we are looking at their eyes; looking at our watches might unintentionally communicate that we are in a hurry to leave and care more about the time than about our patients.

Assessing patients' satisfaction

The easiest and most effective way to assess patients' satisfaction is to ask them for feedback directly, such as through surveys. They can tell us about the strengths of our office and identify areas for improvement. Positive reinforcement encourages us and our staff to continue the aspects of their visit that patients liked. If patients note aspects that they did not like, we should consider it a gift (which is not always easy to do!) and take advantage of their advice to improve the clinic experience for future patients. Patients may not be right about diagnostic or treatment issues, but they are always right about how they perceived how things went.

Research from surveys on patient satisfaction reveals that the single most important factor that determines patients' satisfaction is whether or not they felt they saw a friendly, caring doctor **(Table 3)** (Uhas AA, 2008). How long we keep patients waiting and how much time we spent with them in the examination room are statistically associated with patient satisfaction but only account for a small portion of the variation in satisfaction; almost all the variation in overall patient satisfaction is determined by whether patients *perceive* that we are a friendly, caring doctor. Satisfaction is not determined by how much we care (we care a lot!) but only by patients' perceptions of how much we care.

Factor	Correlation with Patient Satisfaction
Age	0.01
First visit	-0.03
Routine reason for visit	0.04
Male gender	-0.009
Waiting time	-0.13
Time spent with doctor	0.11
Caring attitude and friendliness	0.87

Table 3: Physician-related factors and their correlation with patient satisfaction

There are many ways to conduct surveys. We can distribute a quick, one-page paper survey in the office ourselves. We can hire independent services to administer and analyze surveys or to call or write to patients. The various approaches vary in their ease and cost. One particularly easy and inexpensive way to assess patient satisfaction is an online patient satisfaction survey service, such as the one at www.DrScore.com, founded by one of this book's authors. **(Figure 7)**.

Figure 7: An example of an online patient satisfaction survey at www.DrScore.com. Online surveys are a cheap and easy way to assess patients' satisfaction.

The open comments from patient surveys demonstrate what patients prioritize in their physicians. Dermatologist James Zalla of Florence, Kentucky, shared the open comments patients made about him on a DrScore.com survey **(Table 4)**. Notice that the comments focus far more on friendliness, caring, and bedside manner—which patients can easily judge—than on technical expertise—which is more difficult for patients to assess. Notice that the third comment in Table 4 is from a patient who waited a long time—over one hour!—to be seen by Dr. Zalla. Yet this patient nevertheless rated their visit with Dr. Zalla a 10 out of 10. Patients may not like waiting, but most will gladly do so in order to spend time with what they perceive to be a caring doctor.

1	This was my first visit with Dr. Zalla. He was very thorough in examining me. Since I have a history of skin cancer, he asked me if I use sunscreen regularly and also asked if I have family members who have had skin cancer. Upon answering yes, he gave me two copies of recommended sunscreens. One for me and one for my sister who is not even a patient of his. This shows his great concern for everyone to help prevent skin cancer.
2	Excellent - I go to eight different doctors, but Dr. James and Dr. Mark operate the friendliest, most efficient office. The nurses are all caring, efficient, and friendly.
3	I would have wished to have not been there so long. I got there 10 min early. 40 min after the appointment time, I went to the exam room to wait another 30-plus min. There must be some way to schedule appointments so wait time is not as long.
4	I got to see the doctor; he was patient, kind, and answered all my questions, even though it was for a different issue than when I had made the appt.
5	I was extremely impressed with his kind and concerned demeanor and the time he gave me. He checked me over thoroughly and spent time reviewing my melanoma on my face. I could not get over how kind he was! It was refreshing and gave me confidence in his care.
6	The exam was thorough and the operative procedure was adequately explained. I never felt rushed.
7	He listens, cares, and is very good at what he does. I will remain with him as my doctor.
8	He made me feel comfortable when he first entered the room, and he made sure I understood what he was doing.

9	The staff was extremely courteous and friendly. It was a very pleasant experience.
10	He explains what he is doing and why; he also emphasizes how to protect against further problems.
11	He is friendly and very concerned about his patients.
12	Dr. Zalla gets a 10 out of 10 not just because he is a good doctor, but also because he spends time with me. He does not act rushed when I have questions and is not afraid of a little quiet pause while I absorb info or try to formulate a new question.
13	The office is incredibly professional, pleasant, calm, and well-run. The staff is very nice and helpful. I felt I was in good hands. It was the best doctor's office experience I have ever had! Thanks for not having a TV in the lobby, but a fountain instead.
14	He took his time to explain his answer properly when I asked a question. He also was looking at me as a person and did identify other issues with me that needed treatment. I would recommend him to other people. Thanks.
15	His examination was thorough and candid. He did not rush me through the exam; he was methodical, took the time to explain the condition, and recommended treatment. A welcome break from the assembly line appointments administered by most doctors these days.
16	I have appreciated his conservatism and calm manner as I have visited him over the past eight years or so. He has always given me excellent and timely care.
17	Dr. Zalla is one of the finest physicians I have ever encountered regardless of specialty. His bedside manner and thoroughness are outstanding. A true product of the Mayo method, he is to be commended both as a caregiver and a technically wonderful physician. 10 out of 10, the best.

18	He was very good with all the questions that I asked him. He told me what he was going to do before he did it; this is one of the best visits that I have ever had with a doctor. We needed more doctors like James Zalla.
19	It is too bad there are not more doctors that care about their patients as much as he does! I wish I had gone to see him before the ER visits and family physician visit. His office is beautiful!
20	Dr. Zalla was very through and explained the proper care and prevention and was not in any hurry.
21	Both Dr. Zalla and his assistant, Sue, were courteous, informative, and professional.

Table 4: Patients' comments on their experience with Dr. James Zalla collected from www.DrScore.com

When patients develop positive perceptions of us, they will trust the treatments we prescribe. Indeed, they will not be as scared about the potential side effects that they see on the package insert inside their medication box. They will use their medication correctly and their condition will improve. They will also be far more open to the idea of trying a novel medication because we have built a relationship of trust over time. Besides, they will also be satisfied with their care, and this outcome alone should make our efforts worthwhile.

Chapter 8
Setting the Right Office Visit Context

The halo effect

The halo effect is the tendency for one attribute of a person or object to "spill over" and affect perceptions of other, even unrelated, attributes of that person or object (Davis SA, 2014). For example, attractive people are generally viewed as more intelligent and trustworthy than those who are less attractive. Attractive people receive better grades than unattractive people of the same intelligence and are treated more leniently by the judicial system. In this example, attractiveness confers a "halo" that positively affects people's perceptions of the individual's other attributes.

We can apply the halo effect to promote patient satisfaction. Since most patients are not equipped to assess our clinical skills accurately, they judge us based on our overall appearance and bedside manner. Imagine one clinic with a clean, organized waiting room that offers complimentary coffee, a variety of magazines, courteous staff at the front desk, kind nurses, and a physician wearing a freshly ironed, immaculate white coat. Now imagine another clinic with rude staff, an untidy waiting room, and a disheveled, poorly dressed physician. Although the physician in the second clinic might be highly competent, patients may make judgments based on the poor appearance of the clinic setting and conclude that this office offers substandard care.

The blue vein illusion and the power of context

The power of context to affect our perceptions is illustrated by the apparently blue color of veins. We should know that veins are not blue from "deoxygenated hemoglobin" because we know that blood is red when we draw blood from veins. Our veins cannot be blue. But even knowing that veins cannot be blue and knowing it is only an optical illusion, if we look at our veins, the veins still appear blue **(Figure 8)**. We cannot control the power that context has on our perceptions.

Figure 8: The blue vein illusion. In this figure, line A is the color of the vein, and it is clearly not blue. Square B is the color of the surrounding skin. When line A is seen in the context of square B, the line has a bluish appearance.

Context of the office visit

Setting the right context—maintaining a clean, neatly arranged office, having staff who are friendly and attentive, posting office signs that convey caring and trust, and adhering to a schedule in which patients are seen on time—helps ensure that our patients perceive we care about them. They might even be more willing to overlook negative aspects of their visit if the appearance of our clinic gives the clear impression that we care about them.

One common scenario is that patients might arrive at our office thinking that doctors only care about money. This perception might be reinforced by signs at the reception desk that outline copayment policies, return check policies, and accepted credit cards **(Figure 9)**. Ideally, our office attributes should not be set up to reinforce such biases.

> Your insurance company requires us to collect your co-payment at the time of service.
>
> The Department of Dermatology requires a copy of your Insurance Card at the time of your visit. Please have your card ready when you check in.
>
> We appreciate your co-operation

> OUR PRACTICE CONTINUES TO GROW THROUGH REFERRALS FROM OUR PATIENTS THANK YOU FOR YOUR TRUST AND CONFIDENCE

Figure 9: Office signs. One of these signs provides information on important office policies, while the other does not. Which one will give the patient the impression that we care more about our patients than about money?

In place of too many signs about our offices' financial expectations, we might post a sign that reads, "We appreciate the trust you put in us and are proud to provide you medical care of the highest quality."

Other strategies to convey the right message to our patients and improve the atmosphere of our clinic are outlined below in a checklist format that facilitates audits of the office environment (Rajpara AN, 2012):

Office evaluation checklist

(Reproduced with permission from *The Dermatologist*)

Waiting room

1. Magazines are in good condition.
2. Water and cup dispenser is clean.
3. The trashcan is not next to the water dispenser.
4. Ceiling panels are unstained.
5. The check-in desk is in good condition.
6. Patient fliers are on a bulletin board, not taped to windows.
7. All windowsills are clean.

Clinic hallways

1. Entrance door is well maintained.
2. Nurses' desk is well maintained.
3. Nurses' area is clean.
4. Patient folders are in good condition.

5. Wallpaper is well maintained.
6. No papers are taped to walls or doors.
7. All signs are laminated.
8. Exam room doors are clean.
9. Cryoablation device is not easily accessible to patients.
10. Chart holders on the examination room door are clean.
11. Dry erase boards outside patient rooms are clean.
12. Pictures and frames are in good condition.
13. Hallways are generally clean and free of dust.
14. There are no scuff marks on the floors.

Exam room

1. Wallpaper is well maintained.
2. There are no holes in the walls.
3. There is no writing on the walls.
4. There is no tape left on the walls.
5. No nails are showing in the wall.
6. Plastic information and folder holders are clean.
7. Sinks are clean.
8. Mirrors are clean.
9. Patient chair and footstool are clean.
10. Equipment tray is clean or covered with a clean drape.
11. Trash cans are well maintained.
12. Patient and visitor chairs are well maintained.
13. Coat hangers are well maintained.
14. Door knobs are clean.
15. All cabinets are well maintained.
16. All windowsills are clean.
17. Floors are clean.

Chapter 9
Fostering Patient Accountability

Accountability may be the most underappreciated, critical component to getting patients to take their medication. Accountability is a widely used motivational technique, be it through formal accounting of sales in business to reporting of research progress at weekly laboratory meetings. While there are many reasons why patients are not able to take their medication, fostering accountability can improve patient adherence regardless of the reasons for poor adherence.

We can hold our patients accountable in a number of ways. If we establish a strong physician-patient relationship, our patients will naturally want to please us; they will want to use their medication so as to not let us down. We can also schedule regular follow-up visits to make them accountable for using their medication in anticipation of their office visits.

Parable of the piano teacher

A piano teacher held weekly lessons with her students for eight to 12 weeks, after which time she held a piano recital at which all the students performed. The audience loved the music; all the children sounded terrific. They performed well at the recital because they had practiced every week leading up to the recital.

Another piano teacher, realizing that it was the students' diligence in practicing rather than the weekly visits that had made them play so well, instructed his students, "We are going to hold our recital in eight to 12 weeks, but we are going to forego the weekly lessons. What makes you play well is practicing at home, not the lessons. Just practice every day, and I will see you again at the recital."

This recital, though, sounded terrible. Without the weekly lessons to encourage the students to practice on their own, they did not practice until just days before the recital. The anticipation of the weekly lessons was critically important in holding them accountable for practicing.

School or work assignments

No one, not in any field of human activity, gives a person a new assignment and says, "Work on this project every day. I will meet with you again in 8-12 weeks." No research lab director would say to a bright, industrious student—even a highly motivated one who desires a dermatology residency position—on a summer research rotation, "Here is your project. Work on it every day, and we will meet again at the end of the summer." The only group who takes such an approach is doctors (and our patients are typically not as high-functioning, industrious, and motivated as students who want to get into dermatology!).

The way we practice, the standard way we start patients on a new medication, is set up to fail. Giving patients a medication and telling them, "See you in 8-12 weeks," does not make sense at all. Now, we are not exactly like the piano teacher who gives kids sheet music and says, "Practice every day; see you in 8-12 weeks." No, we are more like a piano teacher who says, "Here is a prescription for some sheet music. Take it to the sheet music store. I do not have any idea what it will cost you. Get the sheet music and practice every day. It may cause a rash, headaches, or diarrhea. But practice every day, and I will see you in 8-12 weeks."

> **Helpful hint: Cancelling a weekly team meeting**
> Our research team meets once a week, at noon on Fridays, at which time we discuss the progress on our projects. If the lab director was called on Monday and was asked to give a lecture out of town on Friday and accepts the invitation, on what day should he let his minions know that the Friday lab meeting is cancelled? He could tell them on Monday; if he did, his minions might not work very hard that week. On the other hand, if he lets the minions know on Thursday night or Friday morning that he is cancelling the meeting, the minions would get in their usual full week of work.

Clinical trials versus real-life practice

Clinical trials often demonstrate how quickly a drug worked, showing statistically significant improvements in outcomes as early as one to two weeks after beginning the drug. The data report displays an elegant curve with data points every two weeks and illustrates how the drug continues to yield improvements over eight to 12 weeks or longer. The Food and Drug Administration approves the drug, and the package insert describes how it is well tolerated and how patients exhibit disease improvement in eight to 12 weeks.

Accordingly, we often prescribe medications and request that our patients return to clinic in eight to 12 weeks **(Figure 10)**. Then, because there were no visits in between and no monitoring of their use of the medication, patients often return reporting that the drug did not work or they that stopped using it because they developed some side effects that they could not tolerate for eight to 12 weeks.

Clinical trials	↓	↓	↓	↓	↓	↓	↓
Week	0	1	2	4	6	8	12
In practice	↑						↑

Figure 10: The frequency of office visits in clinical trials greatly differs compared with that seen in clinical practice. Clinical trials typically include frequent assessment visits. Visits at baseline (week zero) and weeks one, two, four, six, eight and 12 are common. These visits allow researchers to assess the drug's effectiveness over the course of treatment. On the other hand, in the "real world," visits typically occur every 12 weeks. Much like the Heisenberg uncertainty principle in physics, which states that measuring the momentum of a particle changes its momentum, the office visits during a clinical trial change the effectiveness of the drug, making it more effective by improving adherence.

Instead, we can have our patients return for more frequent follow-up visits, much as we do in clinical trials. The higher frequency of office visits in clinical trials indirectly increase adherence, and so we can use a similar strategy to improve adherence in real-life clinical practice. While frequent follow-up visits might not be practical, scheduling the first return visit at week one instead of at week eight may be practical. Approaches other than a return visit—even a planned phone call one week after starting treatment—may be a suitable alternative.

White coat compliance

Mothers of children with acne often tell us, "Doctor, it is so frustrating. You always catch it on a good day. You do not see what it is normally like." Their children's acne is better when they visit us. The reason we seem to catch patients on a good day is the same reason we do not use blood glucose levels to assess control of diabetes at office visits; patients use their medication much better in the few days preceding the visit. Similarly, just as individuals tend to floss their teeth more often prior to visiting the dentist, our patients use their medications just before they come to see us.

When this concept was presented to a neurologist who had specialized in treating Parkinson's disease for over eight years, she explained, "Every day in clinic, the spouses tell me, 'Doctor, it is so frustrating. When you examine him, he moves just fine. But when he is at home, he can barely move at all.'" The neurologist had thought the stress of the examination was somehow altering her patients' neurotransmitters; more likely, the patients simply started taking their medication in anticipation of the visit.

We can use this phenomenon, known as white coat compliance, to hold our patients accountable by scheduling a follow-up visit shortly after starting a new treatment to assess how well the treatment is working (and thereby improve adherence and how well the treatment is working). Dr. Lawrence Feldman of Westminster, Maryland, describes how the concept of white coat compliance changed how he treats acne. Instead of scheduling return visits in six to eight weeks, he has patients come back in two weeks.

"Cyber white coat compliance"

While accountability is a social phenomenon, it does not require direct human contact. For example, in one study, a web-based, weekly reporting intervention doubled adherence to acne treatment in adolescents (Yentzer BA, 2011). Such weekly reporting instills a sense of accountability—essentially cyber or digital white coat compliance. Therefore, if frequent appointments are unfeasible, we ask our patients to call or email us to report how the medication is working, which provides a similar form of accountability.

A Nobel Peace Prize example

In 2006, Muhammad Yunus and Grameen Bank® were awarded the Nobel Peace Prize for their work in using microlending to "create economic and social development from below." Grameen Bank®, founded by Yunus, issues small loans to poor people on favorable terms. The steps to lift people out of poverty, according to Yunus, are to lend them money in amounts which suit them and teach them basic financial principles. Loans may be for as little as $25, although the mean is $200. People can use the loans to purchase a cell phone, chicken, or cow, providing a basis for a small business: a payphone operation, eggs for sale, or milk to sell. Loan repayment rates are in excess of 98%. Microcredit is viewed as a key way to get people out of poverty.

Is merely giving poor people the access to microcredit the solution to poverty? Giving them a loan may be necessary but alone is insufficient. The programs at Grameen Bank® involve more than just giving a small loan. The program also brings together groups of five women who develop business plans and meet weekly with a bank representative to discuss their business development, marketing, and sales efforts. There is enormous social pressure in these groups to market and sell products to repay the loans. The accountability provided by these weekly meetings may be as important for success as the loan itself, just as accountability to the physician may be as important as the prescription for getting patients well.

SECTION 3:
Practicality – Simplicity and Education

Chapter 10: Involving Patients in the Choice of Treatment

Chapter 11: Reducing the Burden of Treatment

Chapter 12: Educating and Providing Instructions

Chapter 13: Helping Patients Remember

Chapter 10
Involving Patients in the Choice of Treatment

Involving patients in the choice of treatment is important because patients often have strong preferences for certain therapies, and those preferences may be different from ours. Typically, the various treatment options for a given dermatologic condition exhibit a wide spectrum in terms of efficacy, safety, and convenience. Some of these issues may be of utmost importance to one patient and of little consequence to another. Some patients prefer a medication that acts rapidly and care little about potential side effects. Others are risk-averse and would rather err on the side of safety. Sometimes otherwise rational patients may display a strong aversion to a particular drug or side effect based on their past experience or the experience of a friend, a very powerful phenomenon that we can use to help patients (we discuss this topic further in Chapter 15: Giving Salient Descriptions).

Patients also differ in how skin disease affects them. A treatment that we view as safe and appropriate might seem far too risky to some patients. Others might deem the same therapy inadequately aggressive. Furthermore, one patient might do anything to avoid a needle (we have ways of dealing with this fear; see Chapter 14: Anchoring), while another might believe an injection is just what he or she needs. Patients' preferences can be widely unpredictable, but they keep our practices interesting.

The Ikea® effect

The Ikea® effect holds that when we put work into obtaining or building something personally, we value it more highly (Davis SA, 2014). The namesake example is that a piece of furniture from Ikea®, which typically requires self-assembly, holds more value than an identical item that comes pre-assembled.

The Ikea® effect suggests that when patients are involved in their treatment plan—when they are making decisions and working with us to solve problems—they become more invested in improving their own health. We can utilize a number of strategies to facilitate this sort of involvement. One approach is to frame treatment options in such a way that the patient adopts the treatment plan as his or her own idea. For instance, we can begin with the open-ended question, "What is important to you in a treatment?" If the patient has difficulty responding, we can progress to a more specific question, allowing the patient to choose from multiple options: "Do you

> **Recommended quote:**
> We can involve patients in selecting a treatment by asking, *"What is important to you in a treatment?"* An appropriate follow-up question is *"Do you prefer a treatment that gets rid of your symptoms as quickly as possible, or one that works slower but has fewer side effects?"*

prefer a treatment that gets rid of your symptoms as quickly as possible, or one that works slower but has fewer side effects?" By facilitating and engaging patients in this dialogue, we can engender a sense of responsibility to adhere to the treatment regimen. This feeling of ownership only becomes possible when the treatment plan is no longer our idea but theirs.

Topical treatments: choosing a vehicle

The age-old dogma for treating skin lesions is "if it is wet, dry it; if it is dry, wet it." We were indoctrinated that conditions that produce dry, scaly lesions should be treated with ointments. We were taught that ointments are inherently more potent than less occlusive vehicles such as creams or lotions because ointments deliver more of the active drug by increasing skin penetration. We were taught to encourage patients with psoriasis and atopic dermatitis to use ointments, even when they are reluctant to do so.

This way of thinking did have some underlying scientific rationale. Many years ago, most ointments did deliver higher amounts of the drug into the skin than did creams or lotions. The occlusive properties of some ointments increase epidermal hydration and reduce barrier function, thereby increasing drug penetration. There may even be anti-inflammatory effects associated with improving epidermal barrier function using an occlusive agent. Nevertheless, *patients will not realize these beneficial effects if they do not apply the product.*

Newer non-ointment preparations, though, are designed to deliver the drug without occluding the skin. Moreover, diseased skin has poor barrier function, so the occlusive properties of an ointment may not be needed. While moisturizing the skin and repairing the epidermal barrier may confer anti-inflammatory effects, they are not essential for controlling inflammation or making skin lesions resolve. Systemic drugs such as cyclosporine and infliximab exert powerful anti-inflammatory effects and can completely clear psoriatic plaques, yet they do not moisturize the skin. Clobetasol, an even more potent anti-inflammatory agent, does not need to be applied in a messy, occlusive vehicle to be effective.

One common method of measuring the potency of a topical corticosteroid is the vasoconstrictor assay. This assay measures the amount of blanching that occurs when the agent is applied: the stronger the steroid, the greater the blanching. The assay assesses two of the three factors that determine the potency of a topical steroid: (1) how potent the drug is in activating corticosteroid receptors and (2) how well the vehicle delivers the drug into the skin. However, the vasoconstrictor assay does not assess a third, often-overlooked factor that affects the potency of topical steroid preparations: whether patients will actually apply the medication. A messy product that demonstrates a high potency in the laboratory setting will not necessarily work well in patients who will not apply a messy product.

Poor adherence has a dramatic effect on the efficacy of topical agents. Steroid ointments, which may be wonderfully potent under the controlled conditions of the vasoconstrictor assay, may show minimal potency in real-life patients who dislike the greasy feeling of an ointment preparation **(Figure 11)**.

Figure 11: Crude coal tar. Crude coal tar is a very effective treatment when applied in the office or hospital setting, but it is far too messy for most patients to use at home. Ointments pose similar issues in many patients.

Fortunately, one of the major advancements in the care of patients with psoriasis was the development of a host of vehicle options for delivering steroids topically. We still have ointments for patients who prefer them, and some patients do like them, as ointments soften hard scale, reduce the pain of fissures, and make scale immediately disappear—the scale does not go away; the change in refraction merely makes it transparent. We now also have creams, foams, gels, lotions, shampoos, sprays, and tapes. For each patient, one of these vehicles will be the best. Which one? The one he or she will actually use.

The characteristics of topical vehicles were assessed in measuring patients' preferences for various vehicles

(Housman TS, 2002). Seven characteristics were identified: ease of application, time required for application, absorption, how it feels to touch, how it smells, how it feels on the skin, and how much it stains. Patients with psoriasis were asked to rate a variety of vehicles—creams, foams, gels, ointments, and solutions—using these criteria. Overall, they preferred the less messy products, particularly foams and solutions, over the more moisturizing vehicles such as ointments.

The notion that patients find ointments messy is not new. Patients have been complaining about ointments for years. Dislike of ointments may explain why so many prescriptions for psoriasis medications went unfilled in Denmark. One approach that has been suggested is to give patients a less messy product to use during the day and an ointment to apply at night, when patients presumably would not mind using the ointment. But when patients were asked to characterize their daytime and nighttime preferences for different vehicles, no significant differences were observed (Housman TS, 2002). In other words, patients generally did not like using the ointment—neither during the day nor at night **(Figure 12)**.

Many patients seem to prefer the new "lighter" vehicles. However, other than asking them directly, there is no *a priori* way to predict what vehicle will be best for a given patient. Ideally, if samples are available, we might have the patient try different vehicles and see which one they prefer. While we have been taught that ointments are best for dry, scaly conditions, this statement is simply not true; if you are not yet convinced of this fact, it may be good to jump ahead to

Chapter 24: Skin Cap for Psoriasis. The best vehicle for a particular patient is the vehicle he or she will actually use.

Figure 12: Patients daytime and nighttime vehicle preferences for various vehicles. Patients strongly preferred using foams and solutions over creams and ointments, regardless of the time of day.

The default option

In research survey studies, patients say they want to know about their options and participate in treatment planning. But in the clinic, patients often ask for clear guidance from us on what treatment to take; they value our opinion about which treatment is best. While we should involve patients in the choice of treatment, we should also guide them, rather than giving them an array of options with no input at all. So many treatment options are available that patients may have a hard time knowing which one to choose. In fact, they may even hesitate to choose any treatment at all, prolonging their suffering with undertreated disease.

Chapter 10 / Involving Patients in the Choice of Treatment

Behavioral scientists studying employees' retirement plans have found that many employees do not sign up for a retirement savings plan, even when employers gave the employees free money in the form of matching funds. This left many employees without an adequate retirement plan. To address the problem, employers began offering employees more retirement plan options. Providing more savings options caused more employees to forego making any retirement contributions! The more complicated the choice, the more employees did not bother to check the box to sign up for retirement savings. Instead, they went with the default option, which was not to sign up at all.

The solution for getting employees to participate was simple: make participating in a basic retirement plan the default option unless the employee had chosen some other plan (or no plan at all). We can use the default option to help patients select and adhere to a single therapy. We can tell them, "The standard approach is drug A, but you could also choose from among drugs X, Y and Z if you prefer."

> **Recommended quote:**
> We can help patients choose the best treatment among many options by stating, "In this situation, the standard approach is drug A, but you have dozens of other choices. Let me get you a few books for you to read that describe these other options in detail."

If we wish to encourage patients to select drug A because we think it is the most appropriate, we might tell them, "In this situation, the standard approach is drug A, but you have dozens of other choices. Let me get you a few books for you to read that describe these other options in detail." Patients are not going to want to read those books. The more difficult, complicated and time-consuming we make it to choose another approach, the more likely patients will go along with the default plan that we suggest. If we want to further drive patients toward the plan we think is best, we can add, "I had a patient whose disease was a lot like yours, and he/she did well on drug A." We will talk more about the value of such anecdotes in Chapter 15: Giving Salient Descriptions.

Chapter 11
Reducing the Burden of Treatment

We should strive to make treatment as easy as possible for our patients and not create needless hurdles. Patients already experience burden from their disease and are busy with their lives. We should avoid treatments that are worse than the disease; we should avoid complicated approaches that patients will not have time to do. Reducing the burden of treatment helps promote adherence and can be achieved via a number of strategies, such as prescribing combination drugs, minimizing complexity, and shortening the treatment interval.

Using combination drugs

Sometimes we want patients to take more than one medication to get the benefit of multiple mechanisms of action to treat their disease. But giving people multiple treatments presents a hurdle to adherence. One helpful approach, commonly used in treating acne or psoriasis, is to prescribe a product that combines two or more medications. In treating acne, we often want patients to use an antiseptic product (perhaps benzoyl peroxide) along with a topical retinoid (such as adapalene). But it is hard enough getting patients with acne to apply a single product. Giving patients more than one product to use complicates the regimen and makes adherence more difficult. In one study, when patients were given one, two, or three or more different prescriptions to fill, 9%, 40%, and 31%, respectively, did not even fill all their prescriptions (Anderson KL, 2015). Giving patients multiple prescriptions reduces primary adherence.

> **Helpful hint: Syncing refills**
> Even going to the pharmacy to pick up refills represents a barrier to adherence. When patients are on multiple medications, their prescriptions may become out of sync, requiring multiple visits to the pharmacy each month to get refills. This is a needless hurdle. Pharmacists can give patients a few extra pills or whatever is needed to get all the prescriptions synced up so that they can get filled at the same time. Use of a mail order pharmacy is another approach to help minimize the burden of being on chronic medical treatment.

Another study found that secondary adherence is higher when patients are given a single product with two active ingredients than when they receive two separate products (Yentzer BA, 2010). Prescribing a product that contains two active agents—such as Epiduo® and Epiduo Forte® (benzoyl peroxide/adapaline), Benzaclin® (clindamycin/benzoyl peroxide), or Veltin® (clindamycin/tretinoin)—makes treating acne less complicated and may improve patients' adherence.

In treating psoriasis, Dovonex® (calcipotriene) ointment works too slowly by itself and thus is best used in combination with a topical steroid. Sequential treatment regimens—initially using both drugs daily, then one on weekdays and the other on weekends, and then one for maintenance—represent an alternative but are overly complicated. Applying two medications at different times of the day increases the chance that patients will miss doses. Moreover, using them at the same time might dilute them, potentially reducing their efficacy. A combination product such as Dovobet®, Taclonex®, or Enstilar® (calcipotriene/betamethasone dipropionate) is useful in this situation. By giving our patients both drugs in a single container for once-daily use, we can make topical therapy for psoriasis less complex and adherence more likely.

Simplifying the treatment regimen

When patients present with refractory skin conditions, we might be eager to add different types of medications, switch to more potent medications, or institute measures that promote occlusion and penetration. Recognizing that treatment failures in dermatology often result from poor adherence, we can see how these efforts might be counterproductive. The solution is not to make the treatment regimen more complicated, but to make it *less* complex.

For example, consider a child whose atopic dermatitis is refractory to emollients and various topical steroids. Adding stronger steroids, oral antihistamines, and wet wraps only makes it more difficult for the parents and child to adhere to treatment. A more reasonable approach would be to limit treatment to a single topical steroid and focus on using that one treatment well. By eliminating ancillary medications, the family can concentrate on applying the one steroid properly, and the child's lesions will clear beautifully in a few days, much as they would if he or she was treated in the hospital.

We also have a tendency to make the treatment of psoriasis more complicated than necessary. Dermatology textbooks recommend keratinolytic agents such as salicylic acid for breaking up psoriatic scales and enhancing the penetration of topical steroids. *Rook's Textbook of Dermatology* claims, "Even the most potent steroid is useless if painted on the surface of thickly heaped-up psoriasis" (Burns T, 2010). Similarly, Habif's *Clinical Dermatology: A Color Guide to Diagnosis and Therapy* states that "scale must be removed first to facilitate penetration of medicine" (Habif TP, 2015). These recommendations, though, contradict the results of studies indicating that thick, scaly plaques exhibit poor barrier function. Furthermore, numerous clinical trials have shown that topical clobetasol alone—without any descaling agent—is highly effective in clearing thick, scaly psoriatic plaques.

Salicylic acid remains a useful agent to reduce hyperkeratosis but is not necessary for permitting steroid penetration, reducing inflammation, or clearing psoriatic plaques. If we can motivate our patients to use their topical steroid, their lesions will improve. Making the regimen more complex by giving separate keratolytic agents may reduce adherence, making the disease all the more "resistant" to treatment. Perhaps *Rook's Textbook of Dermatology* would have been more accurate if it read, "even the most potent steroid is useless if it is not applied." For more on this principle, see Chapter 25: Coral Reef Psoriasis.

Shortening the treatment time horizon

For alcoholics, the heavy burden of quitting alcohol for the rest of their lives is enough to drive them to drink. For this reason, the focus of Alcoholics Anonymous is not on quitting forever, but rather on quitting for a single day—just one day. If the alcoholic is able accomplish this goal and do so consistently, then he or she has essentially quit forever. The task of avoiding alcohol for a single day, one day at a time, appears far less burdensome than quitting forever. Adhering to treatment for chronic skin diseases is not altogether different.

One of the most effective methods of improving adherence is to begin with a short treatment interval. Suggesting that patients use a medication, especially a topical one, several times a day for six to eight weeks represents an extraordinary burden. Imagine being faced with the prospect of applying a topical agent to lesions that are scattered throughout your body twice a day for six to eight weeks. Imagine how difficult this task sounds, as busy as you are already. Now imagine how much worse it would be if you were a parent in charge of applying the medication to your child's skin for those six to eight weeks.

Now consider instead how you would interpret the burden if the doctor had explained, "I am going to ask you to do something very difficult. I would like you to apply the medication to the spots on your skin twice a day. But it is only for the next three days. Then we will see you back in the office and gauge your improvement." Patients will use the medication much better, will have witnessed the benefits of the medication, will have developed a habit of using the medication, and will continue therapy thereafter. In essence, shortening the treatment time horizon lets them see the light at the end of the tunnel. It is a motivating force that strengthens their ability to bear the burden of treatment more easily.

> **Recommended quote:** An effective way to shorten the treatment time horizon is by explaining, *"I am going to ask you to do something very difficult. I would like you to apply the medication to the spots on your skin twice a day. But it is only for the next three days. Then we will see you back in the office and gauge your improvement."*

Switching to an easier treatment regimen

The human brain is not designed to perceive reality in isolation; it is designed to appreciate contrasts. Thus, our perceptions tend to be relative rather than absolute. A sweet cola product, for instance, may taste bitter if we drink it while eating ice cream. A 50° Fahrenheit day might seem warm during the dead of winter but would feel unusually cold during the summer. Our perceptions of touch, sight, smell, and sound are all affected by context.

So too are our perceptions of the burden of treatment. By prescribing our patients a treatment regimen easier than their previous one, they might view their new regimen favorably. We might achieve this end by prescribing a single medication instead of two or by switching to home phototherapy instead of office-based phototherapy. Applying a topical medication once a day is not easy, but it might seem easy to patients who had been trying to do so twice a day. Similarly, using a topical spray is more difficult than taking a pill, but using the spray might seem effortless to patients who had been previously using an ointment.

To make a certain regimen seem easier, patients do not even need to have tried a more difficult treatment. Simply describing some arbitrarily more difficult treatment may be all that is required. We discuss this further in Chapter 14: Anchoring.

Selecting a fast-acting agent

Positive feedback is a strong motivator—when patients see that their medication works, they will be motivated to continue using it. Therefore, a fast-acting agent may be more effective than a slow-acting one. We have a very short window after we prescribe a medication during which our patients adhere to the treatment regimen. Most patients will not patiently wait to see if a slow-acting medication works before they give up on it. When prescribing a slow-acting agent, such as Plaquenil® (hydroxychloroquine) for lupus erythematosus, we advise initially pairing it with a fast-acting agent (for example, topical clobetasol) so that patients see rapid improvement in their disease and are encouraged to continue taking their medications.

Minimizing costs of treatment

Prescribing a medication that patients cannot afford is not a sensible way to encourage adherence. We should prescribe low-cost equivalent medications when available, unless our patients specifically prefer a more expensive product. We can also use our electronic medical record system to auto-populate the following instructions for the pharmacist on our prescriptions: "If the pharmacy offers a similar but less expensive option, feel free to switch to that medication, if the patient wants to." Even generic topical steroids can be very expensive. If we prescribe clobetasol, but the pharmacy offers betamethasone at a lower price, if we and the patient are comfortable with that change, then we can have the pharmacist make the substitution.

> **Recommended quote:**
> To minimize the costs of treatment, we can use the following words in our instructions for the pharmacist that appear on our prescriptions: *"If the pharmacy offers a similar but less expensive option, feel free to switch to that medication, if the patient wants to."*

Chapter 12
Educating and Providing Instructions

It is always a good idea to educate patients about their diagnosis and their medication. Do they know why they were given their medication and how they are supposed to use it? If they understand their disease and how to use the medication, they will be more likely to abide by our recommended treatment plan. To this end, providing patients with information about their condition and with clear instructions for their treatment is critical for maximizing adherence.

Although this information seems basic, it does not always get transmitted to patients. One study conducted in Denmark looked at how often physicians gave patients basic information about the medication they prescribed at the same visit (Storm A, 2009). Shockingly, only two out of three patients were given the diagnosis or told the treatment duration. Only one in four patients were told the effect of the medication, and none were told the potential adverse effects or the cost of the medication. And even when patients were told this information, it was often presented in a way that was not effective. When patients were queried two weeks after the visit, most did not know the diagnosis, the duration of treatment, or how much of the medication to use. We could blame patients for not remembering, but doing so will not help improve our ability to get them well. We have plenty of room for improvement in how we educate our patients.

"Dove™ or Ivory™" versus "Dove™, not Ivory™"

Patients teach us so many lessons. One of the more basic ones came from the mother of a child with atopic dermatitis. Her daughter's atopic dermatitis was flaring. She had already seen another dermatologist for treatment. The child's skin was very dry all over. We asked the mother what soap she had been using to bathe her child; she reported Ivory™ soap. We then asked her whether her prior dermatologist had recommended Ivory™ soap. "Yes," she said. "He told me to use Dove™ or Ivory™."

That sounded odd. Common dermatology practice suggests using a less irritating soap such as Dove™ rather than a harsh, drying one like Ivory™. Would a dermatologist instruct a patient with atopic dermatitis to use "Dove™ or Ivory™?" Not likely. Instead, he or she had almost certainly suggested "Dove™, not Ivory™."

This example underscores the value of written instructions. If patients can misinterpret even the simplest instructions—if they can confuse "Dove™, not Ivory™" with "Dove™ or Ivory™"—imagine how much more confused they must be when we state, for example, "Apply the Dovonex® (calcipotriene) and the Ultravate® (halobetasol) ointments twice a day, such as before work and before bed. Use them for about two weeks or until most of the psoriatic plaques have been cleared. Then, use the Dovonex® twice a day on weekdays and the Ultravate® twice a day on weekends. After some time, see if you can get by with the Dovonex® alone." Can we expect patients to remember all these instructions, much less follow them?

Written instructions

Do not leave adherence to chance. If our instructions are not in writing, all bets are off in terms of what our patients will remember. When prescribing expensive biologic medications, we may tell patients, "Keep the medication refrigerated; do not freeze it." They may get home and wonder, "The doctor said something about refrigeration and freezing. Was it 'Do not freeze?' But why would they have mentioned it if I was not supposed to do it? And if refrigeration is good, freezing must be better." If we want our patients to remember information, we must put it in writing. We cannot expect them to remember what we tell them, especially in the stressful environment of a clinic visit.

Our interactions with patients suffer from the "curse of knowledge." This is a psychological phenomenon in which people who know something cannot properly imagine what it is like not to know. To us, proper use of medications is so ingrained that it is difficult, if not impossible, for us to imagine how foreign those concepts appear to patients. We have to do more than just tell patients what to do. Patients who are hearing new information in the stressful setting of seeing a physician will often forget or, perhaps worse, misremember what they were told. Critical instructions should be given in writing.

Distributing written instructions is easy for specialists who focus on a specific disease or perform a single procedure routinely. Mohs surgeons are particularly good at this. Much like McDonald's®, Mohs surgeons do the same thing over and over again. They are able to give their patients detailed pre- and post-operative instructions that are fully optimized and leave no doubts about what patients can expect and what they should do. General dermatology, though, involves a wide variety of diseases and medications, which makes it more difficult for us to give each patient personalized, written instructions. While the task may be challenging, it is not impossible. With the implementation of electronic medical records, we can now even use smart phrases or templates to construct clearly written, standardized instructions.

Tear-off pads

Dr. Linda Spencer of Crawfordsville, Indiana, suggests using a tear-off sheet of paper to transcribe information for patients. "The pads are in each room," she elaborates. "I started using them at the recommendation of my mother when I opened my practice. I had asked my mother what physicians have done for her that she found helpful over the years, and she said that our family pediatrician used these sorts of pads when I was a kid, and she found it enormously reassuring to have all instructions written down. I have had patients who have kept my instructions over the years to use as a reminder. One patient brought in psoriasis recommendations that I had made back in 1989 that he has kept in his wallet all these years!"

Sticky notes

Dr. Robin Berger of Saint George, Utah, employs a similar approach. "When I see an acne patient, I usually write down their regimen, on a sticky note if possible, so they can put it on the mirror in the bathroom." Besides, placing instructions on the bathroom mirror can serve as a convenient reminder for patients to use their medication. If we pre-print our office name and phone number on the sticky note, we can also do some marketing at the same time.

Avoid writing "use as directed"

"Never write 'use as directed' on any prescription," suggests Dr. Keith Vaughan. "The half-life of their memory of how to use each topical medication is measured in minutes—hours, maybe. And the tube often ends up in a drawer full of other 'use as directed' tubes. Have a medical assistant both verbally explain and provide written directions for unique treatments such as soaks and bleach baths."

Digital resources

Our modern world offers a number of informative digital and printed resources. The American Academy of Dermatology produces easy-to-read brochures. For patients with psoriasis, the educational brochures from the National Psoriasis Foundation may be helpful **(Figure 13)**. We can purchase print copies for our clinics or simply direct patients to the Foundation's website (www.psoriasis.org).

Another digital resource, Vivacare (www.vivacare.com), offers a complete online library that can provide patients with personalized health information about their diagnosis and the recommended treatment plan **(Figure 14)**. Alternatively, we can even create our own online resources for patients. The late Dr. Bill Danby of Manchester, New Hampshire, had developed his own website (www.acnemilk.com) for educating patients about the causes of acne.

Figure 13: The National Psoriasis Foundation brochure on systemic medications. The Foundation offers a wealth of peer-reviewed educational materials. We can hand out these brochures to inform patients about benefits and risks of their medication as well as alternative treatments.

Figure 14: A "prescription" for educational material. Vivacare.com offers an entire online library of educational materials for patients.

Dr. Robert Brodell, formerly of Warren, Ohio, and now chair of dermatology at the University of Mississippi, maintained drawers filled with educational materials in each of his examination rooms. Ensuring that the drawers are organized in the same fashion in each room helped him save time in retrieving them **(Figure 15)**.

Written action plans

The treatment of asthma is complex and involves different medications for maintenance, mild flares, and severe exacerbations. Written action plans represent a powerful tool in treating children with asthma. They encourage parents to evaluate their child's breathing regularly using a spirometer and then to administer specific medications based on the spirometry readings. By outlining clear instructions, written action plans enable parents to administer the proper medication in each scenario.

Figure 15: Pre-printed educational materials. Giving patients printed materials is much easier for a Mohs surgeon than it is for a general dermatologist who manages hundreds of diseases. While challenging, the task is not impossible. Organizing the drawers in the same way in each room can save time.

Treating atopic dermatitis presents similar difficulties. Various agents—moisturizers, low- and medium-potency topical steroids, and non-steroidal topical immunomodulators—are used in different situations, depending on the severity and distribution of the lesions. A written action plan for atopic dermatitis can guide parents in applying the most appropriate agent **(Figure 16)**.

Your Child's Eczema Action Plan

What is eczema?
Eczema, also called atopic dermatitis, is a chronic disease of the skin—meaning it is an ongoing problem. It causes dry, itchy, irritated skin and can be stressful for kids and families. It is not contagious. It sometimes runs in families, but not everyone in the family will have eczema.

Even though there is no cure, there are lots of good ways to control eczema. The BEST thing you can do for eczema is to keep skin moisturized! Kids with eczema have dry skin, and the drier the skin, the more itchy and irritated the skin will be.

Other instructions from your doctor: _____

Here are some tips:
- Bathe daily. Use lukewarm water, 10 minutes or less.
- Use a small amount of mild soap. Choose one that is fragrance free. A liquid or bar is fine. Some that are specially made to be milder include: *Dove, Cetaphil, Purpose, Cerave*
- Pat skin dry—don't rub. Be gentle; rough rubbing can irritate skin.
- Moisturize. This is best done right after bathing, when the skin is still a little wet. Moisturize as needed throughout the rest of the day.
- Choose a moisturizer without fragrance. Here are some examples: *Eucerin cream, Cetaphil cream, Cerave cream, Aquaphor ointment, Vaseline petroleum jelly ointment*
- Choose fragrance-free soaps, moisturizers, & laundry detergent. Don't use dryer sheets; they are too irritating.

What to do in a flare:
Despite good routine care, your child's eczema may still flare. The plan below will tell you what medicines to use to get the flare under control. Don't forget—keep using good routine skin care even during a flare!

What to use during a flare:
_____
_____
_____

USE THESE MEDICINES FOR:
_____

If your child is not better by then, is getting worse at any time, or shows signs of infection (fever, chills, pus, or crusting), call your doctor at _____

CALL US at _____ on: M–T–W–TH–F
Let us know how your child is doing overall.
Next appointment: _____

1. NORMAL/DRY:
Normal skin, a little dry, not itching much if at all.
PLAN:
- Regular skin care routine; moisturize twice daily

2. MILD: Itchy skin with light redness.
PLAN:
- Regular skin care routine, but moisturize a little extra
- HYDROCORTISONE Cream: use once a day until the itching is gone (Use HYDROCORTISONE 2.5% Cream to the face and genitals.)

3. MODERATE: Bad itching that keeps you and/or your child awake at night or causes scratching that leaves marks.
PLAN:
- Regular skin care routine, but moisturize a little extra
- TRIAMCINOLONE 0.1% OINTMENT: use twice a day until the itching is gone (Use HYDROCORTISONE 2.5% Cream to the face and genitals.)

4. SEVERE: Skin that is PAINFUL, RED, CRUSTED, or has PUS. Your child may have a FEVER or CHILLS.
PLAN:
- CALL YOUR DOCTOR TO SCHEDULE AN APPOINTMENT! Your child may have an infection requiring antibiotics.

Figure 16: A modified written action plan for atopic dermatitis. Written action plans are commonly used in asthma to help patients use the proper medication. The treatment plan varies based on the peak airflow measured via spirometry. Similarly, in atopic dermatitis, the intensity of treatment varies according to the severity and distribution of the lesions.

Other tools

Samples

Samples represent an excellent resource that we can utilize to teach our patients how to use their medication. They also facilitate adherence by circumventing the common problem of patients neglecting to fill their prescriptions.

Demonstrations

Some treatments, such as new biologic medications, require patients to perform tasks with which they are not usually familiar. Many patients have no experience with self-injectable medications. One common practice is to show patients how to administer injections using a sample injector and some target object, such as an orange or grapefruit. The injector is placed against the orange, and the button is pressed. Voila! The patient has been taught how to use the medication.

We should not educate our patients this way. Doing so leaves open the possibility that, on the way home, they will stop at the grocery store to purchase some citrus fruit. When they obtain their medication, they may inject it into the fruit and eat the fruit, thinking that was what we had instructed them to do.

Instead, we might have a nurse administer the patient's first injection in the office. Then, we can arrange for the patient to self-administer the next injection under nurse supervision.

Teach-back method

Before we conclude the visit, we can ensure that our patients understand our instructions by applying the teach-back method. This method requires patients to express what they have understood and how they plan to use their medications, while also inviting them to ask any questions. The technique is based on observations that students remember more when they are required to teach others about a topic they recently learned.

Cynical or "pre-educated" patients

Some patients may not take their medication because they do not trust our knowledge on their medical condition. We can reassure these patients by showing them images of the condition from the web.

Other patients may have already educated themselves extensively before coming to see us and may believe they know more than we do. Our natural inclination

> **Recommended quote:**
> When patients proudly tell us that they have read WebMD before coming to see us, we should praise them: *"What a relief! Finally, someone I can talk to at my own level! You would not believe how many patients come here without first taking time to educate themselves about their condition."*

might be to tell these patients how much training we have had, how much experience we have, and how we know what the condition is and what needs to be done for it. Acting on those inclinations is a recipe for escalating conflict. A more effective approach might be to bite our tongues about our own knowledge and experience and instead praise our patients: "What a relief! Finally, someone I can talk to at my own level! You would not believe how many patients come here without first taking time to educate themselves about their condition." By acknowledging and praising their knowledge, they will be far more receptive to our recommendations.

Chapter 13
Helping Patients Remember

Like us, patients are forgetful

There are many times when poor adherence is simply due to patients forgetting to take their medications. This obstacle is common yet understandable given that we often recommend complex regimens that patients may find difficult to follow given their already hectic lives. In many instances, patients may not be in their optimal state of health to remember to take their medications regularly. Furthermore, we are creatures of habit. We go about many of our daily activities without even thinking about them. Starting a new medication is hardly automatic. Until it is built into our routine, it will be routine to miss doses.

It is may beneficial to help our patients develop strategies to remember to take their medications. Unfortunately, there is no single technique or algorithm to identify which type of reminder may work best for a particular patient.

Using the Ikea® effect

We can apply the Ikea® effect to help our patients remember

to use the medications we prescribe. More specifically, we can ask them to come up with a number of options to help them remember to take their medications; even if none of the options work particularly well, the process will promote a sense of involvement. It is important that we elicit these strategies from the patient, rather than imposing them on him or her. For example, instead of us ordering patients to take their medication at the same time each day, we can politely ask them, "At what time of day did you decide to take the medication?" Another strategy might be to ask, "What method do you think would be best to help yourself remember to take your medication: a pill box, an electronic reminder, a sticky note, or a reminder from a family member?" As a result, the Ikea® effect results in patients feeling more involved as they develop their own memory aids, and being more involved will make them more likely to adhere to treatment.

> **Recommended quote:** We should let our patients take the lead in developing reminder systems by asking, *"At what time of day did you decide to take the medication?"* or *"What method do you think would be best to help yourself remember to take your medication: a pill box, an electronic reminder, a sticky note, or a reminder from a family member?"*

Tying treatment to an ongoing behavior

Getting patients to adopt a new behavior is daunting. Getting them to do something along with an existing behavior may be much easier. We can be creative. Simple memory aids and reminders are inexpensive ways to improve adherence. Such aids are commonplace in several spheres of daily living. Dr. Linda Spencer points out, "The key is to tie the treatment to a daily habit." She provides several recommendations:

1. Put the acne medications by the toothbrush to help teenagers remember to use them twice daily.
2. Put a topical antifungal medication under the pillow to remember to apply it nightly.
3. After taking a morning medication dose, put the evening dose in the pocket. At night, empty pockets before changing into pajamas and take the medications that remain.
4. Put the morning medication in or next to the clean, empty coffee pot. Take the medication before filling the coffee pot with water in the morning.

Dr. Spencer also describes how her grandfather handled medication adherence: "Those pill sorters may help but can be difficult to open and may themselves present a barrier to adherence. My grandfather used to put all his medications for the day in a shot glass that he would leave on his kitchen table. At each mealtime, he would obtain the pills he was supposed to take. Whatever was left in the shot glass he would 'chug' at dinner. Yes, it is not the schedule his doctor envisioned, but Grandpa lived to be almost 100 years old."

Dr. Diane Thaler of Sturgeon Bay, Wisconsin, offers similar advice. "I tell people to duct tape the pills or topical medication to their toothpaste," she suggests.

Many approaches can work. One of the authors of this book (Dr. Feldman) developed athlete's foot from doing Tae Kwon Do with his son. The condition required regular use of topical terbinafine to prevent recurrences. Remembering to use the medication was difficult, as Dr. Feldman would only notice the medication after putting his shoes and socks on (and was too lazy to take them off once they were on). Only after putting the medication on top of his socks in the sock drawer would he remember to use it faithfully. Putting the medication in the direct path of life can help make patients use their medication better.

Packaging

What would drug packaging look like if we were trying to discourage patients from taking their medications? We would put medications in bottles of a bland color that blends in with the environment, easy to misplace and overlook, with caps that are difficult to remove. This description sounds a lot like our current medication bottles. It almost seems as though our current pill bottles were created with the goal of deterring patients from taking their medication regularly.

Perhaps more creative packaging designs can promote adherence by helping patients remember the proper dosing of their medications. Consider birth control pill packaging. Birth control pills are very effective but require excellent adherence. Because the pills are packaged into containers indicating which pills are to be taken on which days, adherence is quite good. The containers let patients know whether or not they have taken that day's dose. Similarly, the packaging design for Otezla® (apremilast) helps maximize adherence to a titration dosing schedule **(Figure 17)**. It is designed with three strengths of tablets arranged in a pattern so the patient can follow the correct dosing schedule to titrate up to the daily recommended therapeutic dose. Perhaps all oral medications should be packaged similarly.

Figure 17: The Otezla® (apremilast) initiation pack. This packaging is cleverly designed with three strengths of tablets arranged in a logical pattern based on the time of day, day, and week. Can you imagine how poor adherence would be if patients needed to remember this schedule? © 2014 Celgene Corporation

Devices

A variety of devices may serve as a helpful reminder for patients to use their medication. A variety of innovative products are available at http://www.forgettingthepill.com.

SECTION 4:
Psychology – Behavioral Techniques

Chapter 14: Anchoring
Chapter 15: Giving Salient Descriptions
Chapter 16: Emphasizing Losses Versus Gains
Chapter 17: Framing Risks of Side Effects
Chapter 18: Using Side Effects to Our Advantage

Chapter 14
Anchoring

Anchoring describes our tendency to use one piece of information (the anchor) as a reference point for determining the value of other items (Davis SA, 2014). Most choices and decisions we make are based on an anchor, which serves as a foundation for making sound decisions.

Anchoring represents a common phenomenon that can be used to influence people's decision making. For example, imagine that we are looking to buy a new jacket. We find a nice one normally priced at $495 but today marked down to $95; we would surely buy it. But what if we saw that same jacket and were told, "It normally costs $35, but today the price is $95," there is no way we would buy it. But it is the same jacket that is being sold and the same $95 price in both scenarios. Objectively, other, arbitrary prices should not affect our decision; a computer would evaluate the quality of the jacket and the current price and make a decision accordingly. But the human brain does not view the world so objectively. It considers the anchor, even if someone set the anchor with a completely arbitrary number.

Prescribing injectable biologics

Biologics are very effective for dermatologic diseases such as psoriasis, atopic dermatitis, and hidradenitis suppurativa, but patients are often fearful of injections. A patient who has never received an injectable biologic may subjectively compare taking an injection to not taking one. This comparison can be a frightening hurdle in a biologic-naïve patient who is considering biologic therapy.

This fear of injection is inherently subjective and can be easily modified. An arbitrary anchor can be used to reset patients' expectations and help them overcome their fear of injections. Imagine a scenario in which we wanted to start a monthly-administered biologic such as secukinumab. We might say, "Biologics are like insulin; they are given by injection. You are familiar with how patients with diabetes give themselves insulin injections twice a day, right? Well, this medication is not exactly like insulin—you only need to take the medication once a month." (Lewis DJ, 2017). The hypothetical twice-daily injection serves as an anchor, and the monthly injection suddenly appears as a bargain in terms of the frequency of injections. The objective number of injections does not change, but the patient's perception of that number changes dramatically.

> **Recommended quote:**
> We can use anchoring to reduce the fear associated with injectable biologics by deftly explaining, *"Biologics are like insulin; they are given by injection. You are familiar with how patients with diabetes give themselves insulin injections twice a day, right? Well, this medication is not exactly like insulin—you only need to take the medication once a month."*

In one study, patients with psoriasis who had never received an injectable biologic were randomized into two groups. The first was asked how willing they would be, on a 1 to 10 scale, to receive an injectable biologic for their psoriasis once per month. The intervention group was asked the same question, but was first asked how willing they would be to receive an injection for psoriasis once per day. Participants anchored to a daily biologic were much more willing (median, 7.5) to start a monthly biologic than those not anchored (median, 2.0) to the daily biologic **(Figure 18)** (Oussedik E, 2017).

Figure 18: Anchoring effect: increased patient willingness to consider an injectable biologic. Median willingness to a once-monthly injection in the control and intervention group were 2.0 and 7.5, respectively; the distributions in the two groups differed significantly. Boxes indicate 25th and 75th percentiles; the horizontal line in the box indicates group median; the error bars indicate minimum and maximum values, excluding outliers.

The anchoring phenomenon is familiar in pain perception with biologics. Patients who used prefilled syringes in the past often complain of greater pain with an autoinjector. However, patients starting with an autoinjector who have never received the prefilled syringe rarely complain about pain.

Ethics of anchoring

After we diagnose a patient and offer the available treatment plans, the patient always has at least two options: accept treatment, or refuse treatment. Is it ethical for us to use psychological tools such as anchoring to "nudge" patients toward a particular treatment?

Our utmost responsibility is to ensure that we provide our patients with optimal care. By utilizing anchoring deftly, we can guide patients into making the "right" decision regarding their health. There are always anchors. Patients will evaluate the options we present relative to any existing anchors. Our choice is not whether or not there is an anchor, but rather whether to accept the existing anchor or to choose our own. If a particular anchor is more likely to lead to a better treatment outcome, it would be unethical not to use it.

As long as we are using these psychological tools purely for our patients' benefit, we are acting ethically. Would these tools help us sell more Botox® (botulinum toxin)? Surely they would. Would using them to sell more Botox® be ethical? Now that is another subjective question! If you think using Botox helps patients improve their self-esteem and get the most out of life, you might think that helping the patient choose to receive Botox® is an appropriate, ethical way to practice. If you are only prescribing Botox to help yourself to put your children through college or pay for that second home, these approaches may not be appropriate. How we perceive these subjective issues is largely dependent on their context (see Chapter 8: Setting the Right Office Visit Context for a reminder about the power of context in affecting our perceptions).

Chapter 15
Giving Salient Descriptions

Salience refers to the quality of standing out relative to other objects (Davis SA, 2014). Our mind tends to hold onto ideas that create a vivid picture in our minds. As human beings, we are more emotional than we are rational. The horrible news of a single beheading elicits a much stronger reaction than hearing about tens of thousands of lives lost from automobile accidents or heart disease.

Salient adverse effects

Our extensive training as medical professionals enables us to weigh the risks and benefits of treatment. Thus, it can be frustrating when we have the perfect treatment for a particular patient, only to hear him or her say, "No, I do not want to take that medication. I know someone who got cancer from taking that medication." The side effect may not even be related to the drug, and the person who experienced the side effect may be someone the patient met at a party or at the grocery store. Since many of our new medications can be life-saving and life-changing, patients' tendency to turn down treatment can, in many cases, be downright painful for us as their caregivers.

Oral retinoids, such as isotretinoin, are used for the treatment of nodulocystic acne or acne refractory to other therapies. One publicized adverse effect from the use of isotretinoin is depression, and suicides, although rare, have been reported. Although the use of isotretinoin is closely monitored, the risk of serious depression is very low, and the drug likely prevents far more cases of depression than it causes, the salience of the isolated cases of reported suicides makes some patients reluctant to consider using a highly effective drug.

The same might apply to the interleukin-17 receptor antagonist Siliq® (brodalumab), a drug for psoriasis that was associated with four suicides in clinical trials, resulting in a black-box warning about the risk of suicide. A black-box warning might terrify patients, in spite of the drug's benefits and the high likelihood that the suicides in the study were not caused by the medication. It might actually be better to have black-box warnings outlining the risks of not being treated or being undertreated.

Even when adverse effects are not as dramatic as suicidal ideation, they can be more salient than the benefits of the drug. The patient may have grown accustomed to suffering from the disease, and by comparison, the adverse effects may seem worse than the disease.

Using salience to our advantage

Identifiable victim effect

The identifiable victim effect refers to our tendency to become moved more strongly by the experience of single identifiable victims than by statistics on large numbers of affected individuals. Consider the quote, "A single death is a tragedy; a million deaths are a statistic." Thinking about an identifiable victim moves us because it creates a vivid picture in our minds. Statistics, particularly large numbers, may provide greater scientific detail and information, yet may be wholly unmoving to human emotion.

A salient, emotionally charged anecdote about an adverse effect stands out in patients' minds and is not easily overcome by reason or statistics. As such, reciting data on the low probabilities of rare adverse effects can be a time-consuming, futile exercise that is unlikely to change our patients' opinions. Instead of inundating our skeptical patients with data, we might respond with a salient anecdote or two of our own. We might point out an identifiable victim, such as a celebrity who is

> **Recommended quote:**
> If a patient is scared of a medication because a friend had a bad experience with it, we respond with a salient anecdote of our own. We might say, *"One of our other patients who reminds me of you and had a rash very similar to yours had an excellent response to the medication. In fact, I think I saw that patient in this same examination room."*

doing well on the medication. Or we might state, "One of our other patients who reminds me of you and had a rash very similar to yours had an excellent response to the medication." We might even add, "In fact, I think I saw that patient in this same examination room," to strengthen the perceived relationship. Salience is powerful, and it can work for us too.

Encouraging sunscreen use

We can also put salience to use by changing how we encourage sun protection to prevent skin cancer. When motivating patients to wear a wide-brimmed hat and apply sunscreen regularly, saying, "Use sunscreen so you do not get skin cancer," is often an exercise in futility. Instead, we might tell them, "Make sure you use sunscreen so you do not develop a golf ball-sized, ulcerating, odious, pus-draining tumor on your nose, requiring a major surgery that would involve removing the whole nose, leaving a gaping, dark hole in the center of your face, but it is not so bad because the rubber prostheses they make these days look almost exactly like a normal nose!" While the statement, "use sunscreen so that you do not get skin cancer," also covers this horrible outcome and many others, the more colorful, anecdotal description

> **Recommended quote:** Instead of simply telling patients to use sunscreen to prevent skin cancer, we can apply the principle of salience by telling our patients, *"Make sure you use sunscreen so you do not develop a golf ball-sized, ulcerating, odious, pus-draining tumor on your nose, requiring a major surgery that would involve removing the whole nose, leaving a gaping, dark hole in the center of your face!"*

paints a picture in patients' minds that they will not easily forget.

Reducing tanning bed use

We can also use salience in developing public health cancer prevention strategies. The prospect of developing skin cancer, which usually occurs decades after using tanning beds, may not be salient enough for young tanning bed users. Young people may feel that the short-term benefit of a tan outweighs the long-term risks of skin cancer. However, physical appearance is highly salient, and educational programs that drive home the negative impact of ultraviolet exposure on skin beauty may be more salient and effective (Feldman SR, 2001). Moreover, presenting the effects of tanning as a loss of youthful appearance may be more powerful than explaining that giving up tanning is a great way to prevent skin cancer. We discuss presenting information as losses rather than as gains in the next chapter.

Chapter 16
Emphasizing Losses Versus Gains

Loss aversion describes our preference for avoiding a loss rather than obtaining a gain of comparable size (Davis SA, 2014). This bias can lead to an irrational inconsistency, as our preferences can shift drastically in response to small changes in the presentation of two mathematically identical propositions.

The statin scenario

For instance, imagine a scenario in which we wish to initiate a statin in a patient with hypercholesterolemia. We can expect that controlling the disease with a statin would improve a patient's lifespan by reducing the likelihood of a heart attack or stroke. Assume, hypothetically, that taking the statin would give the patient an expected lifespan of 81 years, whereas not taking it would yield a predicted lifespan of 79 years.

There are two distinct yet mathematically identical ways to present these numbers. We could explain, "If you take this statin, your cholesterol will improve, and you can expect to live two years longer." Alternatively, we could say, "If you do not take this statin, you can expect to die two years earlier."

Although the two propositions are mathematically identical, we perceive them very differently. Living two years longer is a nice bonus, but we absolutely want to avoid dying two years earlier.

Loss aversion in dermatology

Selecting an appropriate treatment

Loss aversion is most apparent in dermatology patients whose disease requires aggressive treatment yet who exhibit a bias toward accepting less treatment. Some patients remain extremely reluctant to use treatments associated with potential adverse effects, even if they result in less suffering than the disease itself. It can be heartbreaking to witness a patient with severe psoriasis who makes the choice to continue suffering by opting for topical therapy instead of considering systemic therapy, out of disproportionate fear of adverse effects.

When a patient articulates these preferences, it may be helpful to forge a dynamic in which the patient chooses between two losses, as opposed to a loss and a gain. Rather than emphasizing the gain of improving the severity of the disease, we might counsel him or her, "This drug can prevent your disease from growing even worse," or "If you do not take this drug, you will continue to suffer from the disease." Faced with the possibility that their disease may progress or cause continued suffering, patients may become more inclined take a risk to avoid the loss.

Encouraging medication use

To encourage patients to use their medication, we can also frame the event as preventing a loss rather than resulting in a gain. In motivating a patient with psoriatic arthritis to take methotrexate, for example, we might avoid saying, "Take this pill so that you maintain joint function." Instead, we might explain, "Take this pill so you do not lose the function of your hands." Although there is no real difference between the two phrases, patients perceive a substantial difference.

> **Recommended quote:** We should phrase outcomes of treatment as losses instead of gains. We explain, *"Take this pill so you do not lose the function of your hands,"* instead of stating, *"Take this pill so that you maintain joint function."*

Promoting proper skin care

Loss aversion can also aid in promoting proper daily skin care. To encourage patients to use sunscreen and avoid tanning beds, we might emphasize the threat of losing the youthful elegance of our skin. Citing the example of a celebrity who lost his or her youthful appearance prematurely due to sun damage would be even more persuasive. This approach is more effective than reciting that sun protection reduces the long-term risk of skin cancer, as events that may occur years later are heavily discounted in perceived importance.

Chapter 17
Framing Risks of Side Effects

Probability bias

Modern life has increased the frequency of situations in which we encounter significantly large or extremely small numbers or probabilities, such as the U.S. deficit stretching into the trillions or new medications conferring a 1-in-1,000 risk of an adverse effect. Our brains are not designed to grasp such large numbers or miniscule fractions. This explains why people play the lottery when there is only a 1-in-100,000,000 chance of winning a fortune. For all practical purposes, a 1-in-100,000,000 chance of winning is essentially zero. More people are struck by lightning... twice! But people think about the possibility of winning, they imagine what it would be like to win, the thoughts fill their cranial cavity, and they act as though there is some significant chance of winning.

Extreme numbers, large or small, lead to probability bias. Probability bias describes our response to situations in which we either magnify a small risk, defined as regressive bias, or mistakenly treat different-sized risks as equal, known as probability neglect (Davis SA, 2014).

Fear of side effects

Humans tend to overrate the importance of rare events, including rare side effects; this is a form of regressive bias. A particular medication's side effect may only occur in one patient out of 1,000, but people's minds tend to focus on that one rather than the other 999. The rare side effect may paralyze patients' willingness to take an otherwise very safe medication.

Since fear alters patients' perception of reality, our job is to calm their fears. If patients are overly afraid of the risks of a particular treatment, we must change their perceptions of these risks if we hope to get them to use their medication. Giving patients a clearer perspective of the risks can help them understand that these risks are well worth it when considering the potential benefits of therapy.

Framing

Framing is our tendency to change how we value a set of options based on our current frame of reference or the frame from which the option is presented. Framing is an important strategy to express small risks in terms that our patients can comprehend.

What "sounds" safer?

A patient once presented to our clinic needing a biologic for his severe psoriasis. However, he would not consider taking any biologic. Ingrained in his mind was the possibility that biologics could cause liver disease, a side effect that he must have had conflated with that of methotrexate. We asked him if he would take the medication if there were only a 1-in-1,000 risk of liver disease. Slamming his hand down on the table, he exclaimed, "No! You are not listening to me! I had a relative who died of cirrhosis. It was a slow, painful death. I would never take it!" We then asked him, "What about another medication in which 99 out of 100 do not get cirrhosis, would you take that?" "Sure, I would take that!" he replied.

What an odd, but typically human way to view these numbers! A drug with which 99 out of 100 have no problem is 10-times riskier than a drug that confers a 1-in-1,000 risk of an adverse event. Nevertheless, stating that "99 out of 100 do not have a problem with the drug" sounds safer than characterizing the risk as 1 out of 1,000. If we are told 99 out of 100 do not have a problem, we picture the 99. If we are told 1 in 1,000 do have a problem, we fixate on that one, especially when the rare outcome is laden with emotion.

Framing risks of biologics

Patients may be terrified by rare adverse events associated with biologics, such as infection or malignancy. Accurately explaining the risks of biologics is a challenge. However, even scarier than quantitative yet accurate descriptions of side effects are ambiguous ones. Vague descriptions may be magnified out of proportion, leading to disproportionate fear of our proposed treatment regimens. If patients hear, "There is a risk of lymphoma," they may behave as if there is a 50-50 risk. Warning patients about a "risk of lymphoma" may be a good way to discourage a patient who does not need a biologic from taking one, even if the biologic has no known risk of lymphoma (inflammatory diseases have a risk of lymphoma, so there is a risk of lymphoma, even if it does not come from the biologic).

> **Recommended quote:** Instead of vague descriptions such as, *"There is a risk of lymphoma,"* we can characterize the risk more accurately: *"The risk of lymphoma from taking the medication is comparable to that of having a fatal accident while driving on a highway."*

Due to our inherent probability biases, it can be difficult for us to use numbers alone in describing the risks of treatments in ways that put those risks into an accurate perspective. For this reason, it is important to communicate the risks in other ways. Emphasizing that the risk of an adverse event is similar to that of a familiar event characterizes it more accurately: "The risk of lymphoma from taking the medication is comparable to that of having a fatal accident while driving on a highway." Visual materials can aid in illustrating the true size of miniscule fractions **(Figure 19)** (Kaminska E, 2013).

```
Lymphoma
Accidents
Lymphoma + TNFi (upper limit)   TB variable screening + TNFi (upper limit)
         ↓                                ↓                                        Heart disease    Cancer
                                        Stroke

├──────┼──────┼──────┼──────┼──────┼──────┼──────┼──────┼──────┤
0%     5%    10%    15%    20%    25%    30%    35%    40%    45%
↑
From least to most:
Lightning strike
MS
TB
TBscreened + TNFi (upper limit)
MVA
MS + TNFi (upper limit)
```

Figure 19: Using visual aids to clarify risks. This graph compares the lifetime risks of tumor necrosis factor (TNF) inhibitors in psoriasis patients to more common benchmarks of risk. Abbreviations: MS, multiple sclerosis; MVA, motor vehicle accidents; TB, tuberculosis; TNFi, TNF inhibitors

The patient who needs a biologic

Imagine if a patient with severe psoriasis were to ask, "Biologics increase the risk of infection, right?" An appropriate and reassuring response might be, "There is a potential risk of infection, but if you look at 100 people who use a biologic for a year, 99 of them do not get an infection." If we are trying to be even more reassuring, we might say, "Because you have so much psoriasis, your immune system is out of whack, and you have about a 1-in-100 chance of developing a serious infection. But if you take this all

> **Recommended quote:** In reassuring patients about the risks of biologics, instead of explaining that there is a 1in-100 chance of infection, we should state, *"If you look at 100 people who use a biologic for a year, 99 of them do not get an infection."*

natural, organic anti-inflammatory agent made in living cells, it will complement your natural healing mechanisms and rebalance your immune system, and 99 times out of 100 you will not get a serious infection. "

If a patient shows a strong preference for no treatment at all to avoid a "risky" drug such as a biologic, we should emphasize that continuing to suffer with the disease is not a risk-free course of action either. Many dermatologic diseases raise the risk of comorbidities, and successful treatment of the disease greatly alleviates this risk. For example, psoriasis is an independent risk factor for the development of obesity, metabolic syndrome, cardiovascular disease, depression, and suicide. In these cases, successful treatment of patients' psoriasis, even with treatments that are not risk-free, might have some potential to reduce patients overall risk of morbidity and mortality, although strong evidence of this benefit is not yet evident.

Decoding patients' language

There are code words in dermatology that signify danger to our patients. One such word is "steroid." We often use the term instead of the far more unwieldy word "glucocorticosteroid." For mothers of children with atopic dermatitis, the seven letters of the word "steroid" may connote "danger." Fear of steroids is common and a common cause of poor adherence (Brown KK, 2006). The word "steroid" may evoke visions of East German female Olympic swimmers with muscular physiques and hairy faces or of Barry Bonds and other steroid-abusing baseball players. No good comes from uttering the word "steroid" to a mother in describing a treatment for her child. Unless we are telling her about a medication that is "not a steroid," we should avoid using the term. We can sense how scary the word "steroid" is to mothers when, after we have prescribed triamcinolone to her child, she immediately asks with trepidation, "Is this a *steroid*?! The last dermatologist wanted me to put a *steroid* on my baby."

When asked a question we do not want to answer, we can use an approach widely used in the U.S. presidential debates: just answer a different question. We do not have to lie and say it is not a steroid. We can just let that question go by, gently put our hand on the mother's shoulder, look her in the eye, and reassure her, "It is a cortisone medication, sort of like over-the-counter hydrocortisone, only a little stronger." If she seems especially afraid, we might even explain, very gently, "This is an all-natural,

> **Recommended quote:**
> Instead of uttering the word "steroid" in front of a fearful mother, we should explain, *"It is a cortisone medication, sort of like over-the-counter hydrocortisone, only a little stronger."* For mothers who are particularly afraid, we can go even further: *"This is an all-natural, organic, gluten-free, topical anti-inflammatory agent made in a peanut-free facility designed to complement your child's natural healing mechanisms and rebalance the immune system and bring it into harmony because we like to take a holistic approach to the management of skin disease in children."*

organic, gluten-free, topical anti-inflammatory agent made in a peanut-free facility designed to complement your child's natural healing mechanisms and rebalance the immune system and bring it into harmony because we like to take a holistic approach to the management of skin disease in children."

In asking about a "steroid," she is really asking, "Is this safe to put on my child?" When we answer, "It is a cortisone medication" or "it is an all-natural, organic, topical anti-inflammatory agent," we are telling her, "Yes, it is safe."

Perceptions of risks

Interestingly, the mere perception of a potential risk, even when no risk actually exists, can strongly influence patients' willingness to use a medication. For example, the information on the package inserts for the topical calcineurin inhibitors Protopic® (tacrolimus) and Elidel® (pimecrolimus) both suggest that their use is associated with an increased risk of lymphoma.

Aside from animal data demonstrating lymphoma formation at a dose 47-times higher than the maximum recommended human dose, there is strong evidence that there is no increased incidence of lymphoma with topical tacrolimus or pimecrolimus (Siegfried EC, 2013). In post-marketing studies, the risk of cancer in patients treated with these medications was *lower* than that in patients who did not receive these agents (Fleischer AB, 2006). Yet the perception of risk has reduced our willingness to prescribe these medications and patients' willingness to use them. Even the non-risk of lymphoma with topical tacrolimus and pimecrolimus remains terrifying!

Chapter 18
Using Side Effects to Our Advantage

Patients can sometimes be terrified of medication side effects. If we tell a mother we are prescribing a "steroid" for her child, she will almost assuredly not apply the medication due to fear of side effects. She will not listen to anything else about the treatment—she will just think about "steroids." The medication is likely to stay in the container, assuming the prescription is even filled. Yet side effects are not all bad. Although they can scare patients, they also represent a powerful tool.

Topical agents that sting

In some cultures, it is commonly believed that if we do not feel a sensation, nothing is happening. Perhaps for this reason some shampoos are even marketed to cause "tingling." For patients who expect to feel a sensation, adding menthol to their topical agent may give them an immediate sense that the medication is working. The sensation created by the menthol may even have direct effects on pruritus.

Some medications prescribed in dermatology do sting without the addition of menthol, particularly alcohol-based solutions applied to broken skin. More specifically, the alcohol-based products prescribed for scalp psoriasis can sting considerably, at least initially. Dr. Richard Fried, of Yardley, Pennsylvania, suggests warning patients, "This medication is so strong it may sting when you first start using it."

Many patients, particularly men adhering to macho ideals, want to "just tough it out" to avoid admitting weakness. We can often turn this maladaptive behavior on its head by challenging them, "This cream may sting. Many men do not have what it takes to use it. Do you think you can do it?"

We can take the challenge of a side effect and turn it into an opportunity to improve patients' adherence to treatment. Whenever there is an expected side effect, it may help to let patients know up front, "You may experience side effect X. In my experience, it is a sign the medication is working." For our scalp psoriasis patients, we can say, "This medication may sting, but that is a sign the medication is working." While this statement is a bit of a stretch, it is nevertheless true—if the medication is causing stinging, the patient is applying it correctly to the scalp (not just to the hair), and if the medication is getting onto the scalp and into the skin, then it is surely working.

> **Recommended quote:**
> For patients with scalp psoriasis who are using alcohol-based products, we can use side effects to advantage by stating, *"This medication may sting. It is a sign the medication is working."*

Other side effects

Some acne therapies, such as oral isotretinoin, may cause dryness. Whether this dryness actually helps improve the acne remains uncertain, but if the patient believes it is associated with improvement, it may encourage them to continue using the medication.

Dr. Adean Kingston of Dallas, Texas suggests perhaps the most innovative use of an adverse effect to improve patient adherence. When prescribing spironolactone to treat acne in women, she informs them, "This drug is a diuretic. In addition to its effect on your acne, you may also notice some weight loss." This statement serves as an excellent example of using an adverse effect to promote adherence. A similar statement could be made when discussing Otezla® (apremilast) for the treatment of psoriasis, as taking apremilast can also be associated with weight loss. More commonly, apremilast is associated with nausea and headaches. We can let patients know that, in our experience, these side effects are a promising sign that the drug is working.

SECTION 5:
Special Considerations

Chapter 19: Patients with Psychiatric Conditions

Chapter 20: Pediatric Patients

Chapter 21: Suddenly Adherent Patients

Chapter 22: The Most Adherence-Resistant Patients

Chapter 19
Patients with Psychiatric Conditions

Psychological factors frequently occur in patients with dermatologic disease and can influence patient adherence. As such, we must routinely screen our patients for psychosocial issues that may affect adherence and attempt to understand how these issues can make adherence difficult for them.

Depression

Depression exacerbates psoriasis. Some dermatologists believe depression affects psoriasis through "psychoneuroimmunologic" mechanisms, pointing to evidence that antidepressants can improve psoriasis. More likely, depression worsens psoriasis by reducing adherence. Patients with depression are less likely to muster the energy or motivation to use their medications. In these patients, antidepressants may improve psoriasis indirectly by improving patients' ability to use their medication.

Stress

Stress commonly exacerbates psoriasis. Psychoneuroimmunologic mechanisms may be at work here as well, but poor adherence provides a simpler explanation for the effect of stress on psoriasis. Under increased stress, patients are less likely to remember to take their medication, and thus adherence worsens.

Personality disorders

Obsessive-compulsive personality disorder

Patients with obsessive-compulsive personality disorder are a dream in terms of adherence. They exhibit rigid conformity to rules and procedures, perfectionism, and excessive orderliness. These patients likely floss their teeth every day. We can rest assured they will use their medication.

Patients with an inclination toward an obsessive-compulsive personality are fairly easy to identify. They often work as accountants, engineers, or architects. During their visit, they may even show us a spreadsheet, meticulously created on Microsoft Excel, listing every medication they have ever tried and categorized using multiple colors.

Not only can we count on obsessive-compulsive patients to use their medication, but we can also can enlist their help in ensuring that others take their medication. Some of our most adherent patients have a spouse with obsessive-compulsive tendencies. For patients who have proven unreliable, we can make their obsessive-compulsive spouse responsible for ensuring they use their medication.

Antisocial personality disorder

Patients with antisocial personality disorder lie at the opposite end of the personality spectrum. Antisocial personality disorder is characterized by a disregard for social rules, societal norms, and cultural codes as well as impulsive behavior and an indifference toward the rights and feelings of others. Patients with this personality disorder will not use their medication and will feel comfortable lying to us about it. These patients need a short adherence leash. We should give them easy-to-use, fast-acting medications. If they fail to respond quickly, it may be best for us to resort to office-administered treatments.

Delusions of parasitosis

One of the most challenging conditions to treat in dermatology is delusions of parasitosis, or Morgellon's disease (Feldman SR, 2016). In this nightmare of a disease, patients describe experiencing the sensation of organisms crawling on their skin, which can cause severe picking and insomnia.

Antipsychotics may prove useful in treating delusions of parasitosis. However, prescribing these medications can be difficult because patients are often reluctant to accept treatments that contradict their disease model, as they believe the disease is caused by parasites, not the mind. Accordingly, when discussing antipsychotics, we should explain, "The parasites seem to be irritating the nerves in your skin and are causing you a lot of itching. We should try a medication to calm down these nerves." We can even explain, "Pesticides are used to kill bugs. Most pesticides work by targeting the nervous system, so we will need to use a medication that works on the nervous system of whatever bugs or worms are there. We cannot use regular insecticides because they are poisonous to humans, too. But we can use medications that work on the nervous system. While these drugs are normally used in psychiatry, we can use them in you to get rid of the bugs." Because patients with delusions of parasitosis usually exhibit poor insight, long-acting depot antipsychotics might be a reasonable treatment in these patients to maximize adherence.

> **Recommended quote:**
> We can broach the topic of starting an antipsychotic by saying, *"Pesticides are used to kill bugs. Most pesticides work by targeting the nervous system, so we will need to use a medication that works on the nervous system of whatever bugs or worms are there. We cannot use regular insecticides because they are poisonous to humans, too. But we can use medications that work on the nervous system. While these drugs are normally used in psychiatry, we can use them in you to get rid of the bugs."*

Chapter 20
Pediatric Patients

Adherence in pediatric patients is a particularly complex issue. For one, we are now working with two distinct audiences—the child and the parents. Even more, these parties tend not cooperate with each other.

As children grow older, they increasingly assume responsibility for adherence. In younger children, problems with adherence usually originate from parents' difficulties in administering the medication, and it may be helpful for us to ask parents about their struggles or proactively provide strategies that avoid potential hurdles. For older children, the problem more often arises from the child rather than from the parent. For example, an adolescent might report having taken medications when, in fact, he or she has not. We must recognize a growing child's role in adherence and address issues pertaining to both the child and the parents.

Young children

Assigning parental responsibility

Medication use in young children is totally dependent on the parents. Pediatric oncology research on adherence to chemotherapy for leukemia show that adherence can be *worse* in two-parent households than in single-parent households (Bhatia S, 2014). What could explain this finding? In single-parent households, it is clear who is responsible for adherence. In two-parent households, each parent thinks the other is in charge, and so there is a diffusion of responsibility. Each parent may think the other will give the child the medication, resulting in no medication being given; alternatively, each parent may feel responsible to give the medication, and medications may be given twice! Therefore, when we are treating children who come from two-parent households, we should ask which parent will be primarily responsible for adherence.

Empowering young children

One mother, a physician, shared her own story about treatment of her son's atopic dermatitis:

> I am a full time anesthesiologist with administrative duties. My son was 12 at the time, a good kid and generally responsible for himself. My son manages his asthma with two medications daily without prompting. He asked to see someone for the dry, itchy skin he had on the inner folds of his elbows. These had turned white and thickened.
>
> Looks like eczema, I thought, and I made an appointment to see our dermatologist, who is my good friend. We saw the dermatologist, got a prescription for triamcinolone ointment, got it filled,

handed it to my son, and I am thinking my job is done. Not a crazy thing to do, given that he manages his asthma with two medications and a rescue inhaler with little input from me.

One month later, we go for our follow-up visit, and his elbows pretty much look the same. He stated that he had lost his triamcinolone three weeks ago while on a cruise with his grandparents and that he did not tell me because he thought I would become irritated. This was personally embarrassing as a mother and a physician to stand in front of my colleague and friend in medicine with my non-compliant son. "How can you possibly expect the eczema to improve if you do not even use the medication? Why are we even here if you lost your medication? This is a waste of everyone's time," I voiced.

I think my dermatologist had seen this movie before. "You do not have to use the triamcinolone," the dermatologist told my son. "Your eczema is not contagious, and it will not kill you. If it really bothers you, have your mom get the medication again and use it when you need it. If it does not bother you, leave it alone. It is really up to you."

Six months have gone by, and my son's eczema is still gone. He uses the triamcinolone on his own schedule. I think it was helpful for him to feel empowered about whether or not he uses it.

Praise and self-monitoring

Praise is cheap, and it can be a strong motivator. Whether we are with our patients or our office staff, we should freely give recognition for good work. Similarly, when patients are improving, we should congratulate them for using their medication correctly.

Praise is particularly valuable in treating conditions in children. They crave recognition and are driven by even the smallest bits of positive reinforcement. Once children are old enough to be involved in their own care, we can administer praise by giving them awards as part of a self-monitoring program.

Sticker charts

The power of sticker charts as a motivator should not be underestimated. If we were to propose using sticker charts in a research study, the human subjects research committee might reject the study on the grounds that sticker charts are overly coercive.

When caring for young children, a sticker chart may be just what we need to get them to take their pill or to apply their topical medication. It can be as simple as drawing a one-week calendar grid with two squares for each day of the week, in addition to purchasing a handful of stickers. We can have the parent give the child a sticker each time they use the medication, up to twice a day **(Figure 20)** (Luersen K, 2012).

Figure 20: A sticker system for improving adherence in children. A preprinted calendar or hastily drawn grid, along with some age- and gender-appropriate stickers, are all that parents need. Few things motivate children as much as the recognition they feel when they receive a sticker rewarding them for their good behavior.

Sticker charts give children a sense of pride and accomplishment while also encouraging continued adherence. Behaviorally speaking, they positively reinforce adherence by pairing a reward with the desired behavior. Moreover, the resulting chart may provide a somewhat reliable record of how well the medication is being used. Developing a sticker chart routine with patients takes merely a few minutes that might otherwise be spent adjusting medication regimens that provide little benefit. Children with atopic dermatitis are a good target population for this intervention, affording them autonomy and allowing them to relish the recognition of their accomplishments.

If we were to design the ideal packaging of triamcinolone for use in young girls with atopic dermatitis, it might come with a medication bottle cap that, when opened, plays music from the movie *Frozen*. Such packaging might make children much more excited about using their medication.

The rebellious teenager with acne

Teenagers are in a transition period between the dependency of childhood and the independence of adulthood. They have a desire to assert their independence. They are also overly concerned about fitting in with their peers. Hormones are raging as part of puberty. These hormones not only make them moody and brittle, but they also cause acne. Of all the places where the acne could appear, it primarily inhabits the face, the area of the body that affects how we perceive ourselves, how others perceive us, and most importantly how we perceive others perceive us.

As if this coalescence of factors was not enough, the lesions on the teenager's face may be more distressing to the parent than to the child. The mother may feel the lesions need to be cleared to assuage her feelings of guilt about the condition. Moreover, her child is transforming into an adult, and sometimes she does not want to accept this reality. She may not be ready to give up control. The interaction between a teenager attempting to achieve independence and a controlling parent usually ends in loud confrontations.

Imagine a teenage boy, sitting on the end of the examination table, with a baseball cap pulled down low over his face. Long and bushy hair protrudes from underneath the cap. Between the cap and the hair, his face is covered by a shadow that obscures even his acne. His mother is sitting on the other side of the room with an angry look on her face. "Tell him to use the medication," she says in an irate, forceful tone. "He is not using it the way you told him!"

Of course he is not using the medication. He is not using it because she is telling him to use it. He wears a hat indoors because it bothers her; moreover, if she is a New York Yankees fan, he may wear a Mets hat. His hair is so long because she wants it short. At every opportunity, the child is attempting to assert independence, even if it means suffering with more acne.

Improving adherence in adolescents

No controlled studies have been performed to assess interventions for poor adherence associated with a controlling mother, but logic dictates asking her to distance herself from the situation. Doing so allows us to assign responsibility to the adolescent, making him accountable over whether or not the acne improves and whether to use the medications or not.

In her review on improving adherence to acne treatment, Dr. Hilary Baldwin offers several suggestions to improve adherence in teenagers with acne (Baldwin HE, 2006):

1. Maximize the quality of the office visit, focusing attention on the patient-physician relationship.
2. Recognize self-conscious patients' need for modesty.
3. Give patients control over their care.
4. Involve patients in the choice of vehicles.

5. Make patients better as soon as possible so that they see that the medication works.
6. Do not waste time pushing ineffective treatments.
7. Recognize patients who do not want to be treated.
8. Educate patients thoroughly and carefully, dealing with anticipated side effects proactively.
9. Confront non-adherence.
10. Examine non-adherent behavior.
11. Create a contract with patients.

Whereas teenagers are highly resistant to overtly strong messages telling them what to do, they desperately seek the acceptance of their peers. For this reason, normative behavior may be a valuable tool. We should advise them, "This medication will give you control over your acne the way other kids have control. It is the one most other teenagers use." We would not tell them, "Most teenagers are not getting better because most of them are not using their medications." Teenagers want to be like other teenagers.

> **Recommended quote:** Because teenagers love to fit in with their peers, we can tell them, "This medication will give you control over your acne the way other kids have control. It is the one most other teenagers use."

One study examined techniques to improve adherence in teenagers with acne (Yentzer BA, 2011). The study found that the group of teenagers whose parents received daily phone calls telling the parents, "Do not forget! Remind your child to use the medication," showed significantly worse rates of adherence than the group that received no daily reminders.

A similar study found that daily text message reminders are ineffective in improving adherence to topical acne medications. Perhaps teenagers perceive the daily reminders as irritating, triggering a sense of resistance and thereby reducing adherence. Conversely, a weekly web survey designed to hold teenagers accountable doubled adherence **(Figure 21)** (Yentzer BA, 2011).

Figure 21: Use of a web-based survey to improve treatment outcomes for teenagers with acne. A web survey can make teenagers more accountable for the use of their medications. Patients who were sent the survey exhibited two-times higher adherence than those who were not sent the survey.

Teenagers, like all patients, need reminders, but they do not like being told what to do. So rather than suggesting that they use a reminder system, we might tell them, "Most teenagers find it helps to have a reminder system. Some put the medication next to their toothbrush, others put a sticky note reminder on their mirror, and whereas others put the medication on their pillow. I do not know which method would work best for you. When you come up with one that works well for you, would you mind sending me a text message to tell me about it? Your approach might help some of my other patients."

Chapter 21
Suddenly Adherent Patients

While improved adherence typically leads to better treatment outcomes, sudden improved adherence in previously non-adherent patients can have unanticipated, serious adverse effects due to excessive drug exposure.

"Resistant" hypertension

When patients reduce the use of their medication without informing us, we may increase the dose of medication or prescribe additional medications to help control the condition. For example, consider patients who appear to have resistant hypertension, defined as having a blood pressure above goal despite the use of at least three optimally dosed antihypertensive medications of different classes. We may prescribe multiple agents at high doses to control the hypertension.

However, the real reason their blood pressure is "resistant" to treatment may be poor adherence. When such a patient is admitted to the hospital for some other medical condition— for example, pneumonia— the intern or hospitalist might write orders for all the anti-hypertensive drugs to be given, and the patient may take all these antihypertensive medications together for the very first time. This sudden increase in adherence may cause severe hypotension that sends the patient to the intensive care unit.

Epilepsy camps

Similar sudden increases in adherence can occur in children with chronic diseases who are sent to a medical camp. For example, consider children with epilepsy who are poorly adherent to their antiepileptic regimen and who, therefore, have breakthrough seizures. Because these children take their medications before the office visit, blood levels will show therapeutic levels. In order to control the breakthrough seizures, a second or third anti-seizure drug may be prescribed, but rarely taken.

Then, when these children attend a summer camp for kids with epilepsy, they may develop toxic drug blood levels. Being at camp may be the first time these kids regularly take the prescribed doses of their antiepileptic medications. Finding children with lethargy and other signs of medication overdose is common in this setting.

Chapter 22
The Most Adherence-Resistant Patients

Some patients are extremely resistant to using their medication. They may be very forgetful. They may be very leery of medication side effects. Others may simply not want to get better due to secondary gain. Nevertheless, we can use certain approaches to assure good adherence in even the most adherence-resistant patients.

Hospitalization

For some patients, the best option may be to relieve them of their responsibility for taking their medications. Self-administered treatments can be substituted with physician-administered treatments. For example, when topical therapy is not working for a localized inflammatory process, the agent is likely not being applied. It is for this reason that atopic dermatitis rapidly improves when the patient receives topical triamcinolone in the hospital. In this case, hospitalization is a very effective, albeit expensive, way to ensure adherence—the medication is applied regularly by the nurses. Home health services may be appropriate for some patients and offer similar benefits.

Office-administered treatments

Hospitalization or home health services, though, are typically not necessary. Indeed, in many cases, the patient can simply come to the office to have the treatment applied.

Topical therapy

For patients with localized psoriasis "resistant" to topical steroids because of poor adherence, we might recommend phototherapy and have our nurse apply the topical agent before each phototherapy session. We could explain to our patients that applying the medication helps the ultraviolet light penetrate the skin more effectively. In clinics without standard phototherapy equipment, we could even apply the topical agent in the office and use a handheld light device, such as a Wood's lamp, to deliver the "phototherapy" treatment. In this scenario, the light itself may be irrelevant; when the patient comes to the clinic, it gives us a chance to apply the topical agent. The plaques will then exhibit very rapid improvement, even when the same topical therapies were ineffective when prescribed for self-administered use.

Methotrexate

If a patient is receiving methotrexate for psoriasis, lichen planus, or another inflammatory disease, and if the medication is not working as expected, do not assume the disease is resistant to the medication; the patient might simply not be taking it. It is hard to blame patients for being terrified of taking their methotrexate at home after we tell them about the potential risks, such as cirrhosis, pancytopenia, and pulmonary fibrosis.

An alternative is to switch the methotrexate from oral administration to weekly intramuscular injection. However, be sure to watch out for adverse effects. If the patient has "failed" 15 mg/week of oral methotrexate because he or she was not using it, a dose of 15 mg/week of intramuscular methotrexate may be too high. In other words, consider reducing the dose when switching from patient-administered to physician-administered treatment. New-onset regimented adherence, in a previously non-adherent patient, can have serious consequences. Refer to the previous chapter, Chapter 21: Suddenly Adherent Patients, for more on this topic.

Biologics

When self-administered biologics seem to be losing their effectiveness, consider the possibility of poor adherence. Changing to a new treatment or complicating the regimen by adding treatments may not be necessary.

Patients with severe psoriasis may benefit from the TNF inhibitor Remicade® (infliximab), which is administered intravenously at infusion centers. However, patients can develop resistance to infliximab for reasons other than poor adherence, such as the formation of anti-infliximab antibodies. For these patients, it may be helpful to add methotrexate in combination with infliximab to reduce the likelihood of developing resistance. If the patient is at high risk for poor adherence, the methotrexate can be given intramuscularly in the office, too.

Other TNF inhibitors, such as Enbrel® (etanercept) and Humira® (adalimumab), are not associated with the same degree of antibody-mediated treatment resistance seen with infliximab. Nevertheless, the efficacy of these agents may also decrease over time, possibly due to antibodies but also possibly due to poor adherence to drug administration or poor handling of the drug. Patients may put the drug in the freezer or, even if they refrigerate the drug, the refrigerator temperature may be set too low (we've seen bottles of water in our refrigerator freeze if kept too close to the coils).

> **Recommended quote:** We can broach the topic of administering self-injectable medications in the office by explaining, *"Sometimes when patients administer the medication themselves in the home, it does not always get to the part of the skin where it works best. For the next few weeks, our nurse will give you the injection."*

Although etanercept and adalimumab are normally patient-administered medications, it may be reasonable to have a nurse administer the medication in the office (Lewis DJ, 2017). We might explain to our patients, "Sometimes when patients administer the medication themselves in the home, it does not always get to the part of the skin where it works best. For the next few weeks, our nurse will give you the injection." Besides, another biologic, Stelara® (ustekinumab), is commonly given as an office-administered injection; better adherence to ustekinumab could be one explanation for the better persistence to ustekinumab treatment when compared with persistence to anti-TNF drugs used for psoriasis (Sandoval LF, 2013).

SECTION 6:
Sample Cases

Chapter 23: Pediatric Atopic Dermatitis

Chapter 24: Skin Cap for Psoriasis

Chapter 25: Coral Reef Psoriasis

Chapter 26: Scalp Psoriasis

Chapter 23
Pediatric Atopic Dermatitis

Atopic dermatitis is very responsive to mid-potency topical steroids such as triamcinolone. Even severe atopic dermatitis rapidly clears with inpatient application of topical steroids. However, many patients have disease "resistant" to triamcinolone prescribed for outpatient use. Such resistance can in many instances be attributed to poor adherence, but patients and their caregivers often remain adamant that the steroid was ineffective, assuring us that they used it correctly.

Poor adherence in atopic dermatitis may be due to a number of factors—complex instructions, lack of trust in us, displeasure with the topical agent vehicle, steroid phobia, and cost of the medication. Nevertheless, simple measures may promote adherence.

Case description

A two-year-old girl came to clinic accompanied by her foster mother reporting a two-year history of unremitting, unrelenting eczema, mostly affecting the extremities but also involving the trunk (Lewis DJ, 2017). The mother, a registered nurse, reported that the lesions had persisted despite applying 0.1% triamcinolone ointment twice daily for nearly two years. Skin examination revealed typical eczematous lesions on the extremities in an extensor distribution. Her disease was particularly severe around the ankles, with overlying crust and excoriations.

The mother, quite convincingly, *insisted* that the triamcinolone ointment had been ineffective. When asked who had been applying it, she reported *she had been applying it personally* on her daughter's skin. She was queried for missed doses, but *she insisted that she had been applying it twice daily*. When asked how much of the medication she had purchased, she described obtaining the recommended amount.

Given her report that the topical triamcinolone had failed, we instructed the mother to apply 0.05% clobetasol ointment twice daily, report how it was working after three days, and subsequently return to applying triamcinolone following the brief course of clobetasol.

The next day, the mother sent us an email message, reporting, "You were absolutely right about the triamcinolone ointment! We were previously told to only use it 'sparingly'...I think I just was not using enough of it for two years....Her eczema looks so much better even after 24 hours!...I will not be filling the prescription for clobetasol. Clearly you were right, and all she needed was a more liberal application of the triamcinolone. I am so glad we came to see you yesterday!"

Case reflection

Shortening the treatment time horizon

Suggesting that our patients apply a topical agent for six to eight weeks, as is often recommended for atopic dermatitis, would place a large perceived treatment burden on the patient or caregiver. On the other hand, encouraging communication within three days of the visit shortens the treatment time horizon. It alleviates the psychological burden associated with long-term adherence, while also fostering accountability during the early stages of treatment. It also enables the patient to witness the rapid benefits of well-used treatment and become assured that this treatment is effective when needed. Perhaps the mother had envisioned the frightening prospect of having to apply a seemingly dangerous "steroid" to her daughter's youthful skin for years. Shortening the treatment time horizon, though, allowed her to focus on the more feasible task of applying the ointment for a mere three days without fear of long-term side effects. As a result, the infant's lesions resolved in a single day after reportedly persisting for nearly two years.

Simplifying the treatment regimen

It is also important to avoid complicating the therapeutic regimen. Adding wet wraps, topical calcineurin inhibitors, penetration enhancers, or more potent topical steroids only makes adherence more difficult. Successful treatment simply involves getting the patient or parent to apply the topical steroid. The most practical approach is to limit treatment to a single steroid to be used once or twice a day for a few days. By eliminating all ancillary medications and emollients from the regimen, the parents can direct their attention entirely to using the topical steroid, after which the atopic dermatitis will clear beautifully in a few days.

Legitimizing the concerns of the parents

While it is important to simplify the treatment regimen, it is equally important to legitimize the parents' concerns. In our case, recommending clobetasol served as a way of affirming that we listened to the mother's report of her experience with the triamcinolone. If we had simply suggested continuing to apply triamcinolone, even after her insistence that it had not been working, she would likely perceive us as insensitive to her concerns. Adherence is markedly lower in atopic dermatitis when mothers perceive that we did not consider their input in designing treatment plans (Fenerty SD, 2013). Since parents are intimately involved in treatment, we must adequately address their concerns if we wish to maximize adherence.

Establishing a "blame-free" environment

One component of a strong doctor-patient relationship involves creating a "blame-free" environment. We must broach the topic of adherence without shaming or accusing patients. In one study, the only circumstance in which questions about adherence were not perceived negatively was if a "de-shaming" communication style was used (Barfod TS, 2006). Assigning culpability for treatment failure is destructive to our relationship with our patients. It engenders feelings of guilt and forces patients to become defensive, reducing the likelihood that they will adhere to our treatment plan. A more effective strategy is to praise parents for being proactive and concerned about their child's health. Such praise builds trust and strengthens the physician-patient relationship.

Chapter 24
Skin Cap for Psoriasis

Exciting news of Skin Cap®

In March 1997, Drs. Dorinda and Walter Shelley wrote in their diary published in *Cutis*, "The big news is Skin Cap, coming out of Spain, now sweeping the country as an over-the-counter spray therapy for psoriasis. Make no mistake about it, it is good. One of our friends said, 'I don't have any psoriasis practice. They all use Skin Cap'....No longer do the patients need steroids inuncted, ingested or injected, and no more methotrexate or PUVA visits. It seems unbelievable that a product not even requiring prescription can be so effective.'" (Shelley WB, 1997).

The product was a zinc pyrithione spray that also contained the detergent sodium laurel sulfate. When the Shelleys gave it to a patient for large psoriatic plaques on the legs, the plaques virtually disappeared one month after using a one-second spray twice a day. They reported on another patient with scalp psoriasis: "Last week one of our patients jumped up when we entered the room to exclaim, 'It's a miracle,' as she showed us the spray can. Her psoriasis of the scalp, which had been modestly improved under our treatment for several months was now gone. It had taken just four days."

Skin Cap® showed unprecedented efficacy. In a study demonstrating its histologic effects on psoriasis (Rowlands CG, 2000), Dr. Bill Danby observed histologic improvement in as little as five hours. Within two weeks nearly all the histologic features of psoriasis had completely resolved. Skin Cap® was a revelation for dermatologists, improving psoriasis that had been resistant to all other previous treatments.

Then came the shocking news that the product actually contained clobetasol propionate (Smith K, 1997; Swanson DL, 2005). To many dermatologists, this news did not make sense. They had been prescribing clobetasol propionate in the form of ointments. The new spray therapy somehow appeared to be more potent than the clobetasol ointment ever was. Given the impression that ointments are more potent than drying sprays, there had to be something else that had made the product so effective.

Why was Skin Cap® so effective?

Some dermatologists thought that it was perhaps due to a higher concentration or greater bioavailability of clobetasol in the Skin Cap® preparation, but studies comparing the delivery of clobetasol with Skin Cap® to that of branded clobetasol preparations revealed no greater penetration with Skin Cap® (Franz TJ, 2003). Others believed that perhaps the zinc in Skin Cap® exhibited a synergistic effect with the clobetasol, an interesting hypothesis given the presence of "zinc fingers" in corticosteroid receptors. One study tested

Chapter 24 / Skin Cap for Psoriasis

this hypothesis in patients with bilaterally symmetric psoriasis lesions (Housman TS, 2003). Lesions on both sides of the body were treated with clobetasol foam; one side also received a spray of zinc pyrithione, and the other side was administered vehicle spray. The side treated with zinc did marginally *worse* than the side not treated with zinc; there was no sign the zinc augmented the effect of topical clobetasol.

What could explain the unparalleled efficacy of Skin Cap®? There were three reasons why Skin Cap® exhibited greater efficacy than the prescribed topical clobetasol products, all of which are related to adherence.

First, the spray formulation of Skin Cap® was easy to use. Although we are often taught to prescribe ointments for psoriasis, many patients are reluctant to apply ointments given their greasy nature. The spray was easier to apply and far less messy, and thus patients were more likely to use it.

Second, patients likely used Skin Cap® regularly because they were less fearful of its adverse effects. When prescribing clobetasol ointment, we often tell patients, "This ointment is the most powerful steroid known to humans. If you use this for more than two weeks, seriously bad things are going to happen to you." These warnings are reinforced by the package insert, which shows even more ominous side effects. Consequently, patients likely did not apply the ointment regularly and returned to the office claiming, "I used the medicine but it did not work. We need to try something else." With Skin Cap®, we essentially told patients something like, "This ointment cannot hurt you. It contains the same ingredient as Head & Shoulders® shampoo." Patients used it regularly, and their psoriasis rapidly improved.

Third, patients likely applied Skin Cap® frequently because they had paid for it themselves. When patients purchase a medication, they are more likely to use it. A similar phenomenon occurs during physician dinner lectures and continuing medical education events. When doctors are not charged a fee when registering in advance, they are less likely to attend the event than if a registration fee, however small, had been charged.

Lessons from Skin Cap

The effectiveness of Skin Cap® illustrates that psoriasis, even its most resistant types, can be cleared quickly when patients use their medication regularly. This finding has been amply demonstrated in research studies with non-moisturizing clobetasol preparations. In these studies, clobetasol spray and foam products are very effective. In trials investigating the efficacy of two different forms of clobetasol—Olux® foam and Clobex® spray—psoriatic plaques are clear or almost clear in 60-80% of patients in two to four weeks (Reid DC, 2005; Beutner K, 2006; Warino L, 2006).

A very large community trial revealed that 80% of plaques cleared or almost cleared with four weeks of using twice-daily clobetasol spray (Lebwohl MG, 2017). This high degree of efficacy was observed in newly diagnosed patients in addition to patients who were previously treated with and resistant to other topical therapies, phototherapy, or systemic therapies. 80% clear or almost clear in one month is more effective than our most effective biologics! More recently, a trial studying twice-daily topical desoximetasone spray showed that it alone can clear or almost clear psoriatic plaques in nearly 40% of patients in four weeks (Saleem MD, 2017).

The efficacy of topical clobetasol when applied as prescribed should not be surprising. Imagine if oral prednisone 1 mg/kg/day were administered for psoriasis. While systemic steroids are not used in psoriasis due to potential adverse effects, the psoriasis would probably clear very quickly. Assuming 100% absorption, no first-pass hepatic metabolism, and uniform drug distribution, the tissue concentration in the skin from a 1 mg/kg dose should be roughly 1 mg/kg or 10^{-6} g per gram of tissue. In contrast, the concentration of topical clobetasol is 0.05%, or 5×10^{-4} g/gm—500 times higher than the 1 mg/kg with oral prednisone—not to mention that clobetasol is many times more potent than prednisone is at activating corticosteroid receptors. Although clobetasol is not fully absorbed, it is applied directly to diseased skin, which exhibits an abnormal barrier function that facilitates penetration. Accordingly, topical clobetasol should be *extraordinarily* effective for localized plaque psoriasis. And it is, but only if patients actually apply it.

Topical clobetasol does not need to be prescribed as an ointment. A topical agent does not necessarily have to moisturize the plaques; after all, methotrexate or biologics can clear psoriasis without moisturizing the lesions. The patient simply needs to apply the clobetasol to areas of diseased skin. If a patient prefers an ointment, then we should prescribe an ointment. But Skin Cap® teaches us that if patients do not want to use an ointment, then a less messy clobetasol product may represent a superior treatment option.

Chapter 25
Coral Reef Psoriasis

Psoriatic plaques assuming the morphology of a coral reef with very thick adherent scale—so-called coral reef, ostraceous, or rupioid psoriasis—may be a sign of resistance to topical therapy. However, poor penetration is not the reason for resistance to treatment. The pattern should alert us that the patient may be non-adherent to treatment.

Case description

A 42-year-old male presented with very thick, scaly psoriatic plaques primarily affecting the knees **(Figure 22)** (Feldman SR, 2008). He had failed multiple topical agents. Treatment with Enbrel® (etanercept) 50 mg twice weekly produced mild, temporary improvement. Oral prednisone had been added briefly but also failed to control the lesions. Several treatment options—oral retinoids, phototherapy, and a variety of topical agents and vehicles—were discussed.

In lieu of prescribing phototherapy or a systemic agent, we gave him a bottle of a non-messy, 0.05% clobetasol propionate spray, instructing him simply to apply it, and nothing else, twice daily. We did not prescribe a descaling agent. We scheduled a return visit in three days.

When he returned, the lesions showed marked improvement, with further improvement after two weeks of use. The patient reported that he had used the spray as directed by itself, finding it much more conducive than the messy ointments that had been prescribed in the past.

Figure 22: Treatment of "coral reef" psoriasis with 0.05% clobetasol propionate spray. Plaques with rock-like, coral reef scale (left-most image). At three days, the lesions showed marked improvement with clobetasol propionate spray twice daily (middle image). After two weeks of continued treatment, the lesions exhibited considerably more improvement (right-most image). [Feldman SR, Brown KL, Heald P. 'Coral reef' psoriasis: a marker of resistance to topical treatment. *J Dermatolog Treat*. 2008;19(5):257-8. Reprinted by permission of the publisher (Taylor & Francis Ltd, http://www.tandf.co.uk/journals)].

Case reflection

The presence of coral reef-like lesions served as a tip-off that his psoriasis had been resistant to treatment because of poor adherence. Patients who allow their plaques to grow this thick are clearly not using their medication. The poor barrier function of even thick psoriatic lesions readily permits penetration of topical steroids, if the medication is actually applied. For these patients, we need to start by making sure they trust us. Then, we must find a vehicle they will actually use, such as a non-messy topical steroid. Finally, we should schedule an early return visit to establish accountability for early adherence.

Moisturizers and descaling agents may offer some benefits in dry, scaly conditions, but they are not necessary for the management of inflammatory conditions. If we were to assume that the lesions were resistant to treatment because of poor penetration, we might devise a complicated regimen involving anti-inflammatory and keratolytic agents. Complicating the treatment regimen, though, reduces adherence, yielding worse outcomes than a simpler regimen. A single topical steroid, without keratolytics or an ointment vehicle, may be sufficient. In our patient, recommending a spray, as opposed to an ointment, made it easier for him to use the steroid. Giving him the medication directly obviated the problem that he might not fill the prescription. Lastly, suggesting that he return in three days shortened the treatment time horizon. After experiencing rapid improvement, his confidence in the medication increased, and thus he continued to use it. He had an excellent outcome, despite being "resistant" to so many other therapies in the past.

Chapter 26
Scalp Psoriasis

Of all the conditions in dermatology, scalp psoriasis is one of the most frustrating disorders, for patients and dermatologists alike. I, Dr. Feldman, began to subspecialize in psoriasis in the early 1990s. While treatment seemed to improve most forms of psoriasis, it always seemed as if scalp psoriasis never got better. Nothing left me feeling more inadequate as a dermatologist than taking care of patients whose scalp psoriasis could not be controlled. Holding conversations with other dermatologists and attending American Academy of Dermatology meetings provided no answers. None of the treatments *en vogue* had worked, including oral antifungal agents, keratolytics, topical steroids in all sorts of vehicles, Dovonex® (calcipotriene) solution, and all sorts of drug combinations including "triple gel therapy"—a mixture of Lidex® (fluocinonide) gel, Keralyt® (salicylic acid) gel, and Estar® (coal tar) gel. For twelve years, the cure for scalp psoriasis had been elusive, and I suffered under a cloud of inadequacy, seeing dozens of patients who were simply not improving.

Then the answer suddenly seemed apparent. I had been invited to present a lecture on scalp psoriasis for patients at a national meeting organized by the National Psoriasis Foundation. The venue was a large room lined with rows and rows of patients with scalp psoriasis. Standing at the podium, I began, "Scalp psoriasis is so frustrating." This introduction was meant to show the audience that they were listening to a caring, empathetic doctor. The entire room of heads nodded in agreement. "It is not just frustrating for patients, but it is also frustrating for us dermatologists, too. We like to see our patients get well, and scalp psoriasis just never seems to get better." Again, the room of heads nodded in agreement. "I think I know why it is not getting better," I explained. The entire audience grew silent with anticipation, their heads peered forward and eyes wide open, eager to hear why scalp psoriasis is so difficult to treat. "Because all of you are not putting the medication on your head."

Across the entire room, everyone's heads dropped to their chests as they let out a sigh of catharsis. "Yes," they thought, "I have not been using the medication, and it feels so good to get it off my chest. I have been lying to my doctor about this for so long. It feels good to finally admit to a doctor that I have not really been using the medication."

Misconceptions about scalp psoriasis

Other explanations have been proposed for why scalp psoriasis is often refractory to treatment. One concept is that patients often scratch their scalp, inducing Koebnerization of their psoriasis. Yet patients scratch other areas of their body, and this scratching does not produce psoriatic plaques in these areas that are as treatment-resistant as scalp psoriasis. Another theory is that the scale of scalp psoriasis inhibits the penetration of topical agents. We should know this is not true. The normal scalp exhibits percutaneous absorption similar to the axilla (Maibach HI, 1973), and diseased skin has poor barrier function. Indeed, clinical trials have demonstrated that rapid relief of scalp psoriasis can be achieved with topical clobetasol without a concomitant keratolytic agent (Jarratt M, 2004; Stein L, 2005). Scalp psoriasis is actually one of the forms of psoriasis most sensitive to topical steroids; scalp psoriasis seems resistant to treatment because patients are "resistant" to applying the medication to their scalp.

A thought experiment

Scalp psoriasis is the mother of all poor adherence problems. Consider what it would take to apply a peanut oil product to your scalp. Imagine yourself in the bathroom trying to use the medication. It takes a considerable amount of time to spread it along your entire pre-moistened scalp, and it may involve some mess depending on where it drips. Imagine putting a shower cap on over the product. Now imagine placing your head on your pillow, sporting that shower cap, and experiencing the unpleasant sensation of your hair bathing in a greasy ointment, all while lying in bed next to your date or significant other. Our lives are so busy already. How many of us would adhere to such a time-consuming, messy, and uncomfortable treatment? If a physician told us to follow this routine for a few months, how many of us would quickly give up, if we ever started at all?

Approaches to improve adherence in scalp psoriasis

Choosing the correct vehicle

We should begin with a single treatment; the more complex the regimen, the more difficult it will be for our patients to adhere to the treatment plan. A fast-acting clobetasol product is ideal. We should select an appropriate vehicle; there are many options—a solution, foam, shampoo, oil, among others—but we should prescribe the one that the patient prefers. Mostly, we prescribe generic clobetasol solution. For some patients, a shampoo-based clobetasol product may be preferred. Since most of them use shampoo anyway, recommending a clobetasol shampoo adds little, if any, burden to their daily routine. It may be hard to believe that a short-contact agent such as a shampoo would suffice for scalp psoriasis, given how treatment-resistant it can be. Nevertheless, clinical studies prove this approach is effective, and many patients find it convenient to use (Jarratt M, 2004).

Shortening the treatment time horizon

Because it is so tedious to apply topical agents to hair-bearing scalp, we should reduce the burden of treatment by limiting the treatment time horizon. We might encourage patients to use the medication twice a day for a mere three days. In a recent study, seven patients applied clobetasol lotion to their scalp twice daily for seven days and received phone calls three days after beginning treatment (Rajabi-Estarabadi A, 2017);

six of seven patients were satisfied with the results. Scalp psoriasis clears very quickly with clobetasol, as we learned from Skin Cap®: "'It's a miracle,' ... Her psoriasis of the scalp, which had been modestly improved under our treatment for several months, was now gone. It had taken just four days."

Speaking in the most caring, and empathetic voice possible and with a caring hand on their shoulder, we might express to our patients, "We know it is going to be difficult. We know it is going to be time-consuming. We need you to apply the medication twice a day. But it is only for three days. Come back to the office in three days, and we will see how you are doing. Now it may sting; in my experience, the stinging is a sign that it is working." If the patient lives far away or is too busy to return, we can provide them with our phone number, again expressing our concern for them and asking them to call in three days to report their progress. Implementing a short duration of treatment encourages patients to use the medication, and giving them our phone number engenders trust that further facilitates adherence. It would be much as if the dentist told them, "I am really worried about your gums. Floss your teeth twice a day, and I will see you back here in the office in three days." Patients would floss more during those three days than they might in an entire month!

Simplifying the treatment regimen

One patient had visited the office reporting that her scalp psoriasis had become resistant to three forms of clobetasol therapy—solution, foam and shampoo—simultaneously. Rather than adding yet another medication, we recommended that she focus solely on using the shampoo. We instructed her to apply it twice a day for three days and then call us to report her results. A bit peeved, she asked, "Do you not understand? I am already using that medication, and it does not work." We expressed our understanding and explained that the other two agents might have been working "at cross purposes" with the shampoo. We then asked her to trust us and advised her again simply to use the shampoo for three days. She called back in three days, overjoyed that the scalp lesions had essentially vanished. Had the other two medications been working at cross purposes with the shampoo? They were, in a sense, because the complexity of her original regimen made adherence nearly impossible.

Recruiting a friend or partner

Scalp psoriasis is very difficult for our patients to treat by themselves. Women's hair may have as much as 60 times more surface area than their scalp, so most of the topical agent likely ends up on their hair unless they are extremely careful. One patient remarked that she could only get the medication on her scalp if she had an assistant apply it. In many ways, applying topical therapy for scalp psoriasis is akin to getting our hair colored. The hair is separated down to the scalp, and one row of medication is applied. Hair is successively shifted over, exposing another row of scalp, and the medication is applied again. Following this process for the entire scalp requires two individuals. We might tell our patients, "You have so much hair that you could not possibly apply the medication on your own, so have someone else help you." Every patient loves to be told they have a lot of hair, and this complement strengthens the patient/physician relationship. Furthermore, involving two people—one with the disease and another who applies the medication—doubles the odds that at least one of them exhibits the obsessive-compulsive traits that facilitate effective use of the medication.

Concluding thoughts

Witnessing a patient with treatment-resistant scalp psoriasis rapidly improve is one of the most gratifying aspects of dermatology. Once we understand that scalp psoriasis is refractory because of poor adherence, we can help our patients' lesions improve quickly and easily.

SECTION 7:
Final Thoughts

Chapter 27: Poor Adherence Is Not All Bad
Chapter 28: Conclusions

Chapter 27

Poor Adherence Is Not All Bad

Poor adherence is ubiquitous in dermatology and remains a common cause of treatment failure and frustration among both physicians and patients. Nevertheless, poor adherence is not all bad. One of the best aspects of poor adherence is that it limits the adverse effects of treatment.

Potent topical corticosteroids such as clobetasol or betamethasone are commonly prescribed in dermatology and can induce cutaneous atrophy. It is a wonder that adverse effects occur so rarely—or perhaps it should not be a wonder. The main reason we do not see these adverse effects very frequently is poor adherence.

It is difficult enough to counsel patients to take pills for a week. Getting patients to apply topical agents for long-term management of chronic skin disease represents an even more daunting challenge. Even when their skin disease is intensely bothersome, they may not use their medication. The vast majority of patients stop using their medication as their disease improves. In this sense, poor adherence represents a natural technique for limiting the adverse effects of topical agents.

There are exceptions, though, such as obsessive-compulsive patients who might continue using topical medications long after they actually need them. Atrophy commonly occurs in areas with thin, delicate skin, such as the face, axilla, or groin. However, atrophy can also occur in areas where patients are obsessed about their disease— for example, the shins in women— to the extent that they continue applying topical steroids after the lesions have already resolved and flattened. Indeed, if the induration and scale has disappeared, but the patient continues to use topical steroids for residual macular erythema, atrophy may occur. This outcome is certainly unusual, and such a finding would be incredibly rare in scalp psoriasis.

Chapter 28
Conclusions

Being cynical about patients' adherence is likely a positive thing. We might consider changing what we call "self-administered" medications to "self non-administered" medications. The costs of poor adherence and patient-proclaimed treatment failures are significant. Frequent clinic visits and half-full bottles of medications add to the direct costs of chronic skin diseases such as atopic dermatitis and psoriasis.

Who is at fault for poor adherence? We are. We have so many tools to get patients to use their medications, but we often fail to apply them. At the foundation, we should establish a physician-patient relationship that engenders trust, and we should incorporate some form of accountability into the treatment plan. Our treatment approaches should be simple and tailored to our individual patient's preferences. On top of that, we can use a variety of psychological tools to further encourage good adherence.

Dermatology is an interesting field on many levels. For those new to the field, the number of diseases is formidable. The wide array of treatments we use adds another layer of complexity to the management of skin diseases. Yet within a few years, we become adept at making the right diagnosis and choosing the appropriate treatment within milliseconds of seeing the rash. Fortunately, our patients provide a bottomless wealth of novelty and challenges.

The obstacles associated with patient adherence make dermatology a more challenging field. It is incredibly fun when we consider what we have to do to get patients to use their medications. There is no single approach that will work for all of us. Patient adherence is very complex and is influenced by a myriad of factors. Figuring out how to get our patients to use the medications we prescribe is partly art, partly science, and all fun.

Nevertheless, we can make certain generalizations. First, we ought to assume that patients will likely experience difficulty using their medications regularly. For this reason, we must ensure that patients recognize that we are trustworthy, caring physicians committed to helping them get well. We should also establish accountability, especially early in the treatment period when patients are developing the habit of taking the medication. We should involve patients in the choice of treatment, proposing treatment regimens and delivery systems with which they are comfortable. We should avoid overstating the risks of adverse events and instead use them to our advantage by letting patients know that they are a sign the drug is working. We should also formulate treatment plans conducive to rapid improvement. Once they see that the medication works, they will continue using it. Otherwise, the patient will observe limited initial improvement and will be more likely to give up on the medication altogether.

New drug development offers great promise for our field. But we already have medications in our armamentarium that can benefit the overwhelming majority of patients. Helping them use the agents we prescribe may be more important than developing the next innovative therapy. Whether we are the first dermatologist to see the patient or the sixth, we must remember that our responsibilities include more than simply making the right diagnosis and prescribing the right therapy. We must also do our best to get patients to use their medications.

References

Ali SM, Brodell RT, Balkrishnan R, Feldman SR. Poor adherence to treatments: a fundamental principle of dermatology. *Arch Dermatol.* 2007 Jul;143(7):912-5.

Alinia H, Feldman SR. Assessing medication adherence using indirect self-report. *JAMA Dermatol.* 2014;150(8):813-4.

Anderson KL, Dothard EH, Huang KE, Feldman SR. Frequency of Primary Nonadherence to Acne Treatment. *JAMA Dermatol.* 2015 Jun;151(6):623-6.

Baldwin HE. Tricks for improving compliance with acne treatment. *Dermatol Ther.* 2006 Jul-Aug;19(4):224-36.

Balkrishnan R, Carroll CL, Camacho FT, Feldman SR. Electronic monitoring of medication adherence in skin disease: results of a pilot study. *J Am Acad Dermatol.* 2003 Oct;49(4):651-4.

Balkrishnan R. The importance of medication adherence in improving chronic-disease related outcomes: what we know and what we need to further know. *Med Care.* 2005 Jun;43(6):517-20.

Barankin B. *Dermographies: Autobiographies in Dermatology, Volume 2.* Nova Scotia, Canada: Community Books, 2006.

Barfod TS, Hecht FM, Rubow C, Gerstoft J. Physicians' communication with patients about adherence to HIV medication in San Francisco and Copenhagen: a qualitative study using Grounded Theory. *BMC Health Serv Res.* 2006;6:154.

Beutner K, Chakrabarty A, Lemke S, Yu K. An intra-individual randomized safety and efficacy comparison of clobetasol propionate 0.05% spray and its vehicle in the treatment of plaque psoriasis. *J Drugs Dermatol.* 2006 Apr;5(4):357-60.

Bhatia S, Landier W, Hageman L, Kim H, Chen Y, Crews KR, Evans WE, Bostrom B, Casillas J, Dickens DS, Maloney KW, Neglia JP, Ravindranath Y, Ritchey AK, Wong FL, Relling MV. 6MP adherence in a multiracial cohort of children with acute lymphoblastic leukemia: a Children's Oncology Group study. *Blood.* 2014 Oct 9;124(15):2345-53.

Brown KK, Rehmus WE, Kimball AB. Determining the relative importance of patient motivations for nonadherence to topical corticosteroid therapy in psoriasis. *J Am Acad Dermatol.* 2006 Oct;55(4):607-13.

Burns T, Breathnach S, Cox N, Griffiths C. *Rook's Textbook of Dermatology*, 8th Ed. Hoboken, NJ: Wiley-Blackwell, 2010.

Carroll CL, Feldman SR, Camacho FT, Manuel JC, Balkrishnan R. Adherence to topical therapy decreases during the course of an 8-week psoriasis clinical trial: commonly used methods of measuring adherence to topical therapy overestimate actual use. *J Am Acad Dermatol.* 2004 Aug;51(2):212-6.

Carroll CL, Clarke J, Camacho F, Balkrishnan R, Feldman SR. Topical tacrolimus ointment combined with 6% salicylic acid gel for plaque psoriasis treatment. *Arch Dermatol.* 2005 Jan;141(1):43-6.

Davis SA, Feldman SR. Using Hawthorne effects to improve adherence in clinical practice: lessons from clinical trials. *JAMA Dermatol.* 2013 Apr;149(4):490-1.

Davis SA, Feldman SR. An Illustrated Dictionary of Behavioral Economics for Healthcare Professionals. CreateSpace, North Charleston, SC, 2014.

Devine F, Edwards T, Feldman SR. Barriers to treatment: Describing them from a different perspective. *Patient Prefer Adherence.* 2017 Nov. Accepted.

Feldman SR, Dempsey JR, Grummer S, Chen JG, Fleischer AB. Implications of a utility model for ultraviolet exposure behavior. *J Am Acad Dermatol.* 2001 Nov;45(5):718-22.

Uhas AA, Camacho FT, Feldman SR, Balkrishnan R. The Relationship Between Physician Friendliness and Caring, and Patient Satisfaction: Findings from an Internet-Based Survey. *Patient.* 2008 Apr 1;1(2):91-6.

Feldman SR, Camacho FT, Krejci-Manwaring J, Carroll CL, Balkrishnan R. Adherence to topical therapy increases around the time of office visits. *J Am Acad Dermatol.* 2007 Jul;57(1):81-3.

References

Feldman SR. Effectiveness of clobetasol propionate spray 0.05% added to other stable treatments: Add-on therapy in the COBRA trial. *Cutis.* 2007 Nov;80(5 Suppl):20-8.

Feldman SR, Brown KL, Heald P. 'Coral reef' psoriasis: a marker of resistance to topical treatment. *J Dermatolog Treat.* 2008;19(5):257-8.

Feldman SR. Advances in and hope for the treatment of parasitosis. *J Dermatolog Treat.* 2016;27(3):197.

Fenerty SD, O'Neill JL, Gustafson CJ, Feldman SR. Maternal adherence factors in the treatment of pediatric atopic dermatitis. *JAMA Dermatol.* 2013;149(2):229-231.

Fleischer AB Jr. Black box warning for topical calcineurin inhibitors and the death of common sense. *Dermatol Online J.* 2006 Oct 31;12(6):2.

Franz TJ, Lehman PA, Feldman SR, Spellman MC. Bioavailability of clobetasol propionate in different vehicles. *Skin Pharmacol Appl Skin Physiol.* 2003 Jul-Aug;16(4):212-6.

Habif TP. *Clinical Dermatology: A Color Guide to Diagnosis and Therapy*, 5th Ed. Maryland Heights, MO: Mosby, 2009

Housman TS, Mellen BG, Rapp SR, Fleischer AB Jr, Feldman SR. Patients with psoriasis prefer solution and foam vehicles: a quantitative assessment of vehicle preference. *Cutis.* 2002 Dec;70(6):327-32.

Housman TS, Keil KA, Mellen BG, McCarty MA, Fleischer AB Jr, Feldman SR. The use of 0.25% zinc pyrithione spray does not enhance the efficacy of clobetasol propionate 0.05% foam in the treatment of psoriasis. *J Am Acad Dermatol.* 2003 Jul;49(1):79-82.

Jarratt M, Breneman D, Gottlieb AB, Poulin Y, Liu Y, Foley V. Clobetasol propionate shampoo 0.05%: a new option to treat patients with moderate to severe scalp psoriasis. *J Drugs Dermatol.* 2004 Jul-Aug;3(4):367-73.

Kaminska E, Patel I, Dabade TS, Chang J, Qureshi AA, O'Neill JL, Balkrishnan R, Feldman SR. Comparing the lifetime risks of TNF-alpha inhibitor use to common benchmarks of risk. *J Dermatolog Treat.* 2013 Apr;24(2):101-6.

Krejci-Manwaring J, McCarty MA, Camacho F, Carroll CL, Johnson K, Manuel J, Balkrishnan R, Hartle J, Fleischer A Jr, Feldman SR. Adherence with topical treatment is poor compared with adherence with oral agents: implications for effective clinical use of topical agents. *J Am Acad Dermatol.* 2006 May;54(5 Suppl):S235-6.

Krejci-Manwaring J, Tusa MG, Carroll C, Camacho F, Kaur M, Carr D, Fleischer AB Jr, Balkrishnan R, Feldman SR. Stealth monitoring of adherence to topical medication: adherence is very poor in children with atopic dermatitis. *J Am Acad Dermatol.* 2007 Feb;56(2):211-6.

Krejci-Manwaring J, Johnson KP, McCarty MA, Carroll CL, Hartle J, Manuel J, Balkrishnan R, Fleischer A Jr, Feldman SR. Comparison of different compliance behaviors in a clinical trial. *Cutis.* 2007 May;79(5):379-81.

Lebwohl M, Colon LE. The evolving role of topical treatments in adjunctive therapy for moderate to severe plaque psoriasis. *Cutis.* 2007 Nov;80(5 Suppl):29-40.

Lewis DJ, Cardwell LA, Feldman SR. Applying behavioural economics to psoriasis treatment: interventions to improve patient adherence to biologics. *J Eur Acad Dermatol Venereol.* 2017 Aug. [Epub ahead of print].

Lewis DJ, Feldman SR. Rapid, successful treatment of atopic dermatitis recalcitrant to topical corticosteroids. *Pediatr Dermatol.* 2017 Oct. In press.

Luersen K, Davis SA, Kaplan SG, Abel TD, Winchester WW, Feldman SR. Sticker charts: a method for improving adherence to treatment of chronic diseases in children. *Pediatr Dermatol.* 2012 Jul-Aug;29(4):403-8.

Maibach HI, Stoughton RB. Topical corticosteroids. *Med Clin North Am.* 1973 Sep;57(5):1253-64.

Marks VJ, Hutchison R, Todd M. Service excellence in dermatology. *Semin Cutan Med Surg.* 2004 Sep;23(3):207-12.

Nelms H. *Magic and Showmanship: A Handbook for Conjurers.* Mineola, NY: Dover Publications, Inc, 1969.

Oussedik E, Cardwell LA, Patel NU, Onikoyi O, Feldman SR. An Anchoring-Based Intervention to Increase Patient Willingness to Use Injectable Medication in Psoriasis. *JAMA Dermatol.* 2017 Sep;153(9):932-934.

Rajabi-Estarabadi A, Hasanzadeh H, Taheri A, Feldman SR, Firooz A. The efficacy of short-term clobetasol lotion in the treatment of scalp psoriasis. *J Dermatolog Treat.* 2017 Jul. [Epub ahead of print].

Rajpara AN, Landis ET, Feldman SR. Office Evaluation: Gaining a Fresh Perspective. *The Dermatologist.* 2012 May; 20(5).

Reid DC, Kimball AB. Clobetasol propionate foam in the treatment of psoriasis. *Expert Opin Pharmacother.* 2005 Aug;6(10):1735-40.

Richards HL, Fortune DG, O'Sullivan TM, Main CJ, Griffiths CE. Patients with psoriasis and their compliance with medication. *J Am Acad Dermatol.* 1999 Oct;41(4):581-3.

Rowlands CG, Danby FW. Histopathology of psoriasis treated with zinc pyrithione. *Am J Dermatopathol.* 2000 Jun;22(3):272-6.

Rubin BK. What does it mean when a patient says, "my asthma medication is not working?" *Chest.* 2004 Sep;126(3):972-81.

Sandoval LF, Huang KE, Feldman SR. Adherence to ustekinumab in psoriasis patients. *J Drugs Dermatol*. 2013 Oct;12(10):1090-2.

Shelley W, Shelley D. A dermatologic diary. Portrait of a practice. *Cutis*. 1997 Apr;59(4):181-2.

Smith K. Skin Cap: what have we learned, and when did we learn it? *Dermatol Online J*. 1997 Dec;3(2):11c.

Stein L. Clinical studies of a new vehicle formulation for topical corticosteroids in the treatment of psoriasis. *J Am Acad Dermatol*. 2005 Jul;53(1 Suppl 1):S39-49.

Storm A, Andersen SE, Benfeldt E, Serup J. One in 3 prescriptions are never redeemed: primary nonadherence in an outpatient clinic. *J Am Acad Dermatol*. 2008 Jul;59(1):27-33.

Storm A, Benfeldt E, Andersen SE, Andersen J. Basic drug information given by physicians is deficient, and patients' knowledge low. *J Dermatolog Treat*. 2009;20(4):190-3.

Swanson DL, Pittelkow MR, Benson LM, Hawkridge AM, Muddiman DC. Déjà vu all over again: skin cap still contains a high-potency glucocorticosteroid. *Arch Dermatol*. 2005 Jun;141(6):801-3.

Warino L, Balkrishnan R, Feldman SR. Clobetasol propionate for psoriasis: are ointments really more potent? *J Drugs Dermatol*. 2006 Jun;5(6):527-32.

Yentzer BA, Hick J, Williams L, Inabinet R, Wilson R, Camacho FT, Russell GB, Feldman SR. Adherence to a topical regimen of 5-fluorouracil, 0.5%, cream for the treatment of actinic keratoses. *Arch Dermatol.* 2009 Feb;145(2):203-5.

Yentzer BA, Camacho FT, Young T, Fountain JM, Clark AR, Feldman SR. Good adherence and early efficacy using desonide hydrogel for atopic dermatitis: results from a program addressing patient compliance. *J Drugs Dermatol.* 2010 Apr;9(4):324-9.

Yentzer BA, Ade RA, Fountain JM, Clark AR, Taylor SL, Fleischer AB Jr, Feldman SR. Simplifying regimens promotes greater adherence and outcomes with topical acne medications: a randomized controlled trial. *Cutis.* 2010 Aug;86(2):103-8.

Yentzer BA, Gosnell AL, Clark AR, Pearce DJ, Balkrishnan R, Camacho FT, Young TA, Fountain JM, Fleischer AB Jr, Colón LE, Johnson LA, Preston N, Feldman SR. A randomized controlled pilot study of strategies to increase adherence in teenagers with acne vulgaris. *J Am Acad Dermatol.* 2011 Apr;64(4):793-5.

Yentzer BA, Wood AA, Sagransky MJ, O'Neill JL, Clark AR, Williams LL, Feldman SR. An Internet-based survey and improvement of acne treatment outcomes. *Arch Dermatol.* 2011 Oct;147(10):1223-4.

Zaghloul SS, Goodfield MJ. Objective assessment of compliance with psoriasis treatment. *Arch Dermatol.* 2004 Apr;140(4):408-14.

Made in the USA
Middletown, DE
12 September 2025